Acute and Chronic Renal Failure

Michael Boulton-Jones, MB, B.CHIR, MRCP
Consultant Physician, Royal Infirmary, Glasgow

Published,
in association with
UPDATE PUBLICATIONS LTD., by

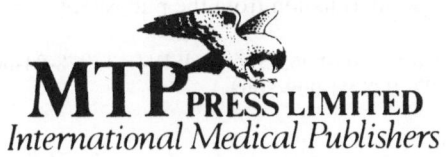

MTP PRESS LIMITED
International Medical Publishers

Published,
in association with
Update Publications Ltd., by

MTP Press Limited
Falcon House
Lancaster, England

Copyright © 1981 MTP Press Limited
Softcover reprint of the hardcover 1st edition 1981
First published 1981

ISBN-13: 978-94-009-8065-5   e-ISBN-13: 978-94-009-8063-1
DOI: 10.1007/ 978-94-009-8063-1

Contents

Acute Renal Failure

1. Introduction

Renal function fails abruptly in a bewildering variety of clinical situations which lack any common clinical pattern. This makes it impossible to define acute renal failure in the same way as heart failure or liver failure. Even oliguria, the commonest sign, is not invariably present. As a result, the detection of acute renal failure

Table 1. Causes of acute renal failure.

Acute tubular necrosis	Ischaemic type
	Nephrotoxic type
Cortical necrosis	

Hepatorenal syndrome

Occlusion of main renal arteries

Occlusion of arterioles
Malignant hypertension
Haemolytic uraemic syndrome
Thrombotic thrombocytopenic purpura
Postpartum nephrosclerosis

Acute glomerulonephritis
Post-streptococcal
'Crescentic' nephritis ⎫
Necrotizing glomerulitis ⎬ idiopathic with systemic diseases

Renal vein thrombosis

Obstruction
Uric acid crystals
Stones
Tumours—benign and malignant
Fibrosis
Strictures

(ARF) depends on biochemical tests, which are fortunately simple to perform and are commonly available.

However, the clinician has to think of the possibility in order to test the diagnosis. Frequently, patients are admitted to a renal unit from medical, surgical or gynaecological wards where the development of ARF has gone unrecognized, either because the relevant investigation has not been performed or because the result has been overlooked. This happens because ARF occurs in patients with complex problems which themselves demand considerable attention, and it is easy to overlook a comparatively rare, if important, complication.

ARF is best denoted biochemically by a rapidly rising serum creatinine. There are several causes of this (Table 1), but the three main groups are acute tubular necrosis, diseases affecting the renal parenchyma or renal microvasculature, and obstruction of the urinary tract.

2. Acute Tubular Necrosis

The term acute tubular necrosis was introduced in 1950 to describe the clinical syndrome of ARF following a great variety of clinical events (Table 2). On pathological examination the kid-

Table 2. Clinical 'causes' of ATN.

Surgical causes
Complications of surgery
  Haemorrhage
  Depletion of extracellular fluid volume
  Sepsis
  Obstructive jaundice
Pancreatitis

Traumatic causes
Extensive trauma
Sepsis
Shock
Burns—fluid depletion and infection

Obstetric causes
Criminal abortion—overwhelming infection
Severe pre-eclampsia and eclampsia
Antipartum haemorrhage
Amniotic fluid embolus
Intrauterine death

Medical causes
Nephrotoxins
Septicaemia
Leptospirosis
Viral infections (coxsackie and influenza)
Low cardiac output

Mismatched blood transfusions

neys are enlarged and the parenchyma bulges through the cut capsule. The cortex appears pale, but the medulla is darker than usual. Histologically, the glomeruli are normal but the tubules show some dilatation and flattening of their cells. Casts may be present in the distal tubules, and interstitial oedema is sometimes prominent. Regeneration of tubular cells, with frequent mitoses, is seen during recovery.

Pathophysiological studies highlight three clinical situations in which ATN develops (see Figure 1): the first two lead to a primary reduction in renal blood flow, and the third is the response to a circulating nephrotoxin. The first two are by far the most common

Table 3. Causes of 'ischaemic' ATN.

Loss of circulating volume
Haemorrhage
Plasma—through burns
Saline—by diarrhoea and vomiting
Inadequate fluid replacement
Septicaemia—by venous pooling

Decreased cardiac output
Following open heart surgery
Severe sudden left ventricular dysfunction

---

and their causes are summarized in Table 3. The clinical picture is dominated by the cause of the reduction in renal blood flow, and the renal failure itself may produce few symptoms or signs. It is thus impossible to give a clinical description which would apply to every patient; clearly there is little similarity between the patient who develops ATN following a severe myocardial infarction and one who collapses in labour as a result of amniotic fluid embolism. The variety of clinical presentations and the subsequent management of these acutely ill patients is perhaps the main clinical challenge and the attraction of this branch of medicine.

Nephrotoxic ATN provides a more uniform clinical picture, and the list of nephrotoxins and the clinical situations in which they occur is given in the Table 4.

Table 4. Nephrotoxic ATN.

Haemoglobinuria
Mismatched blood transfusion
Haemolytic crisis
March haemoglobinuria

Myoglobinuria
Crush injuries
Viral infections—coxsackie B, influenza
Seizures
Strenuous exercise
Hyperpyrexia

Drugs
Paracetamol
Cephaloridine (+frusemide)
Colistin
Amphotericin B
Isoniazid
Polymixin
Gentamicin
Neomycin
Quinine

Chemicals
Ethylene glycol
Carbon tetrachloride
Trichlorethylene
Heavy metals (particularly mercuric chloride)
Phosphorus
Paraquat
Potassium chlorate
Phenol

Clinical Approach

It is customary to describe clinical syndromes in terms of symptoms, signs, investigation and management. This is difficult in the context of ARF and, therefore, it is more appropriate to describe the situation as seen by a nephrologist asked to visit a patient who is likely to develop or may already have developed ATN. When doing this, he has four aims in mind:

1. To determine the facts from every possible source.

2. To see if he can prevent the development of ATN in patients

particularly at risk. These include patients undergoing major surgery, those who have a low cardiac output for whatever reason, and anyone who has a septicaemia or who has been exposed to a nephrotoxin. Whatever the cause, the quicker it is corrected, the less likely it is that ATN will develop. It is also probable that a diuretic (either mannitol or frusemide) given to the patient once the extracellular volume has been restored to normal, in sufficient doses to produce a urine volume of 50 ml/hr, may prevent or retard deterioration in renal function in some patients.

3. To correct any reversible factors that have precipitated renal failure, if it has already occurred.

4. To protect the patient from the dangerous consequences of renal failure.

Examination of the notes and observations taken during the patient's stay in hospital will often point to the probable cause of the development of renal failure. Thus the patient may have had an operation and then suffered a secondary haemorrhage leading to a period of hypotension, all of which has been carefully documented and appears to be sufficient cause for subsequent events. However, other patients with exactly the same clinical course fail to develop renal failure, and yet others, whose pulse and blood pressure have hardly deviated from normal, develop severe oliguria and renal failure. It is therefore obvious that unidentified factors are sometimes crucial in the aetiology of ATN. The clinician can only look for known risk factors and seek to correct them, hoping that if this is done early enough, renal failure can be averted.

Hyperkalaemia

The correction of hyperkalaemia will not of itself improve renal function, but its appearance is a dangerous development because it produces few symptoms before fatal arrhythmias intervene. It should be one of the first considerations.

There are only two ways to make the diagnosis: by frequent measurements of the serum potassium concentration, and by ECG monitoring. The first abnormality to develop on the ECG is

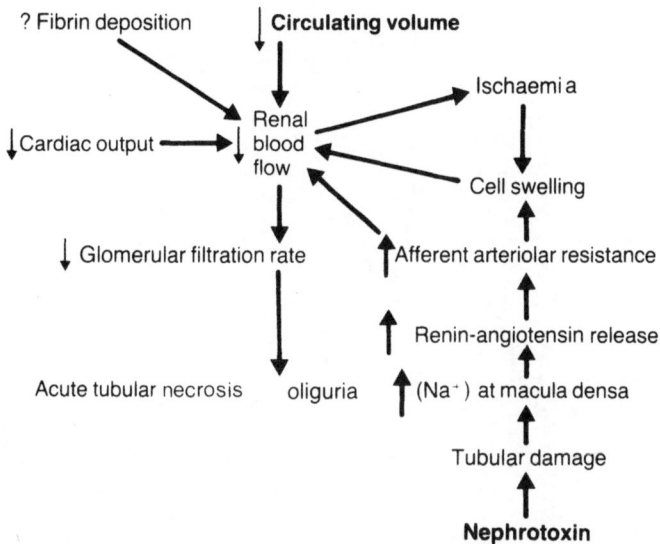

Figure 1. *Postulated pathophysiology of acute tubular necrosis. The three common starting points are decreased circulating volume, decreased cardiac output and a nephrotoxin.*

the prolongation of the PR interval followed by peaking of the T waves and widening of the QRS complexes (Figure 2). P waves then disappear and severe bradycardia and/or ventricular fibrillation develop. The exact concentration of potassium at which these changes occur varies from patient to patient, with the serum calcium and with other factors (e.g. whether the patient is receiving digitalis or has ischaemic heart disease). Any potassium concentration above 6.5 mmol/l should be regarded as dangerous and specific treatment given.

Decreased Circulating Volume

Decreased circulating volume may occur as a result of haemorrhage (which may be occult), extensive burns, persistent vomiting and/or diarrhoea, or through insufficient fluid replacement post-

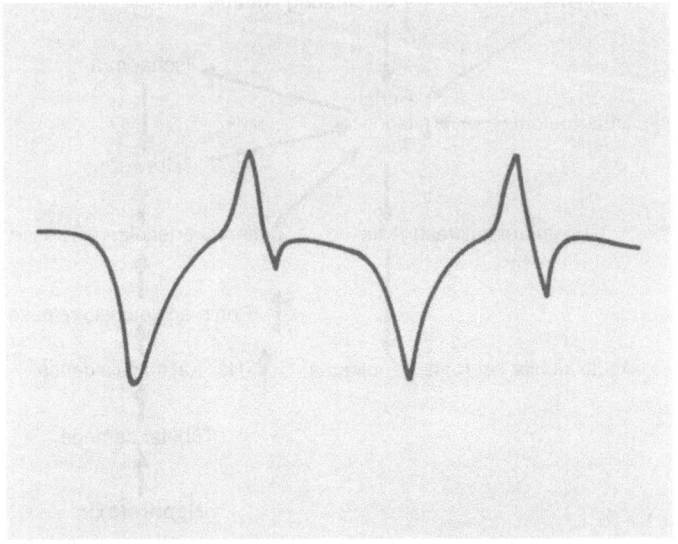

Figure 2. *Changes of hyperkalaemia (K^+ = 9.0 mmol/l). Note the tall T waves and wide QRS complexes. The rhythm is nodal and no P waves are visible.*

operatively. A careful history or examination of the fluid chart may help to determine how much fluid has been lost, but both are notoriously inaccurate. Therefore, the clinical examination is of paramount importance, but unfortunately the signs are non-specific and sometimes difficult to interpret.

Tachycardia and hypotension, initially postural, are cardinal signs, although the latter usually appears late, except in the elderly. The patient may complain of thirst, have cold hands and collapsed veins. Decreased tissue turgor is sometimes helpful, but is difficult to interpret in elderly patients. A dry tongue is of no help in the patient who mouth breathes, and many clinicians find it impossible to draw sensible conclusions from palpation of eyeballs. Conversely, the presence of oedema does not exclude the possibility of a reduced circulating volume; the two may coexist in patients with hypoalbuminaemia or rapid changes in fluid balance or in the elderly. The lack of good clinical signs means that even an experienced clinician can have difficulty in deciding fluid management in some patients. A well placed central venous pressure line can be of considerable help, but is liable to introduce infection and may be misread by inexperienced staff; CVP readings should not be believed if they are contrary to all the other clinical evidence. In the final analysis therapeutic trials of fluid replacement may be necessary, and if improvement of the patient's condition results, further fluid is justified. Frequent clinical examination is necessary so that errors can be quickly corrected. The foregoing cautionary tales should not obscure the fact that in most patients, the diagnosis can be made quite easily as all the evidence is consistent.

Fluid Overload

Fluid overload is found less commonly on the first visit to the patient and usually results from the administration of excess fluid to oliguric patients. Many of the signs are the same as those of congestive cardiac failure—tachycardia, raised jugular venous pressure, oedema, crackles at the lung bases and an extra heart sound, but the patient's extremities are usually warm and the veins dilated. Oedema alone is not necessarily a sign of fluid overload.

Infection

Infection is the main cause of acute tubular necrosis in 5 to 10 per cent of patients, and a contributing factor in a further 25 per cent. More than half the patients who have ATN develop some infection during their illness. The common sites of infection are the urinary and respiratory tracts, wounds and the bloodstream. Pelvic infection (often clostridial) is invariable in patients developing ATN after a criminal abortion. The introduction of the Abortion Act (1967) in the UK dramatically reduced the number of patients presenting with this form of ATN and, in terms of preventive medicine, the Act must be considered a success. Extensive burns inevitably become infected, often with resistant pseudomonas, which is almost impossible to eradicate, and contributes to the horrifying mortality of this subgroup of patients. Reduced fluid intake, mouth breathing and poor oral hygiene predispose to oral infections (Plate 1) sometimes leading to parotitis, a most painful and distressing infection which saps the patient's morale and will to get better, but which has been largely eradicated by proper nursing care.

The typical signs of infection are usually present in patients with ATN, but are sometimes modified; thus lack of fever does not necessarily exclude infection, and neutrophilia is sometimes present when no infection can be found. It is therefore important to culture routinely and persistently blood, sputum, urine and drainage from any wounds. Aerobic and anaerobic cultures should be performed on all specimens. Indirect evidence of infection may be the finding of disseminated intravascular coagulation (Plate 2). A routine coagulation screen is therefore important for this and other reasons. The management of infection is vital to the survival of the patient, as it remains the commonest cause of death.

Bleeding

Patients presenting with uncomplicated ARF have normal values for prothrombin time, partial thromboplastin test with kaolin (PTTK) and thrombin time. Platelet counts are usually also normal, although platelet function can be shown to be deranged by in vitro tests. This may be the reason that patients with ATN bruise easily. Gastrointestinal haemorrhage occurs more commonly in patients with ATN, and there are many reasons for this which have nothing to do with the platelet defect, e.g. hypergastrinaemia, stress, the presence of nasogastric tubes and impaired wound healing. The threat of haemorrhage increases the danger of haemodialysis which requires that the patient's blood be heparinized—at least while it is extracorporeal. For this reason it is a feared complication of ARF and a common cause of death.

Drug Therapy

Most patients who develop ATN in hospital will be receiving drugs when first seen by the nephrologist. Each drug should be reviewed as to both its potential toxic effect on the kidney and its metabolism and route of excretion. Potentially nephrotoxic drugs are listed in Table 4; some drug combinations, e.g. cephaloridin and frusemide, are more toxic than either drug used alone. These preparations should obviously be avoided unless there is a clear indication for their use and no alternative is readily available.

There is one major exception to this rule. Gentamicin is given to patients with ATN more often than any other antibiotic, despite its proven nephrotoxicity in animals. This aminoglycoside, like all others, is excreted unchanged by the kidney, and therefore has to be given in carefully controlled doses, because there is little difference between the therapeutic and toxic levels. The penicillins are also mainly excreted by the kidney, but are relatively non-toxic. They can be given in normal doses, except in the treatment of subacute bacterial endocarditis (SBE) in the uraemic patient, as 12–20 megaunits of benzylpenicillin (the dose normally used in the treatment of SBE) may cause confusion and convulsions. Table 5 includes further examples of the modification of drug therapy required in uraemic patients.

At this stage the clinician should have decided whether the patient has suffered an insult capable of causing ATN and whether that diagnosis requires further proof. He should have identified the reversible factors and be ready to make decisions about further investigation and management.

Investigations

Three groups of investigations are required in the management of patients with ATN (Table 6):

1. Those required to prove the diagnosis of ATN. This is not always necessary as often no other cause for renal failure is likely. There are three ways of confirming the diagnosis:
(a) Urine/plasma osmolality ratio.
(b) High dose intravenous urogram (IVU).
(c) Renal biopsy.

2. Those required for the management of any patient with ATN as summarized in Table 6.

Table 5. Dosage modification of more commonly used drugs for different degrees of renal function impairment (Sharpstone 1977).

	Dose interval (hours) in categories of impaired renal function				Dialysable		Comment (BC=measure blood concentration in severe renal failure)
	>70* None	30–70 Mild	10–30 Moderate	<10 Severe	Haemodialysis	Peritoneal dialysis	
Antibacterial agents							
Benzylpenicillin	8	8	8	12	+	?	BC in 'massive' therapy
Ampicillin	6	6	8	12	+	–	
Cloxacillin	6	6	6	6	–	?	
Carbenicillin	4	4	8	12	+	–	
Tetracycline	6	Avoid	Avoid	Avoid	–	–	Exacerbates uraemia
Doxycycline	24	24	24	24	–	–	No use for urine inf.
Cephaloridine	6	12	Avoid	Avoid	+	+	Potentially nephro-toxic
Cephalexin	6	6	8–12	24–48	+	+	
Cephalothin	6	6	8	12–24	+	+	
Cephazolin	8	12	16	24	?	–	
Cephradine	6	12	24	48	?	?	
Chloramphenicol	6	6	Avoid	Avoid	–	–	Metabolites may be toxic
Co-trimoxazole	12	12	24	24–48	+	?	
Colistin	12	24	48	72	+	+	BC
Gentamicin	8	12	24	48–72	+	–	BC
Streptomycin	12	24	48	72	+	+	BC
Kanamycin	8	24	48	72	+	+	BC
Lincomycin	6	6	6	8	–	–	
Sodium fusidate	8	8	8	8	?	?	
Sulphadimidine	6	6	6	12	?	?	
Nitrofurantoin	6	Avoid	Avoid	Avoid	+	?	Insufficient urine concentration
Para-aminosalicylic acid	12	12	Avoid	Avoid	+	?	
Isoniazid	12	12	12	12	+	+	
Rifampicin	24	24	24	24	?	?	
Ethambutol	24	24	36	48	+	+	

Drug								Comment
Antifungal agents								
Amphotericin	24	24	24	36	−	−	?	Nephrotoxic
Flucytosine	6	8	12–24	24–72	+	+	+	BC
Hypnotics and tranquillizers								
Phenobarbitone	12	12	12	24	+	+	+	
Short and medium acting barbiturates	8	8	8	8	−	−	−	
Diazepam	8	8	8	8	−	−	?	
Chlordiazepoxide	8	8	12	24	−	−	?	
Phenothiazines	8	8	12	18	−	−	−	
Antidepressants								
Tricyclics	8	8	8	8	−	−	+	
Lithium carbonate	8	8	Avoid	Avoid	+	+	+	
Antihistamines								
Chlorpheniramine	6	6	6	6	?	?	?	
Diphenhydramine	6	6	8	12	−	−	−	
Anticonvulsants								
Diphenylhydantoin	8	8	8	8	+	+	?	
Primidone	8	8	12	24	+	+	?	
Trimethadione	8	8	12	24	?	?	?	
Cardiovascular drugs and antihypertensives								
Digoxin	24	36	48	72	−	−	−	
Propranolol	8	8	8	8	−	−	?	
Methyldopa	8	8	12	16	+	+	+	
Guanethidine	24	24	36	48	?	+	?	
Hydrallazine	8	8	8	8	−	−	−	
Lignocaine	Bolus or infusion 4	Un-changed 4	Un-changed 6	Un-changed 8	?	?	?	
Procainamide	4	4	6	8	+	+	?	BC
Immunosuppressive agents								
Corticosteroids	Various	Unchanged	Unchanged	Unchanged	?	?	?	Exacerbate uraemia
Azathioprine	24	24	24	36	+	+	?	
Cyclophosphamide	24	24	36	48	+	+	?	
Antidiabetic agents								
Chlorpropamide	24	36	Avoid	Avoid	?	?	?	
Tolbutamide	8	8	12	12	?	?	?	
Phenformin	8	8	8	Avoid	?	?	?	
Acetohexamide	12	24	Avoid	Avoid	?	?	?	

+ = Yes; − = No; * = creatinine clearance in ml/min.

Table 6. Routine investigation of patients with ATN.

Blood
Sodium ⎫
Potassium
Chloride
Bicarbonate
Urea
Creatinine ⎬ Usually daily
Glucose
Haemoglobin
White cell count
Platelet
Blood gases ⎭
Osmolality
Coagulation screen

Urine
Sodium
Urea
Osmolality

Culture
Blood
Urine
Wound discharge
Sputum
Tracheostomy site

Radiography
CXR
IVU

Weight
If possible

3. Those required for the treatment of the underlying condition which led to ATN. This will not be discussed further.

Urine/Plasma Osmolality Ratio

Urine/plasma osmolality ratio is easily measured. In patients with dehydration and normal renal function, this ratio will be greater than 1.7, but in patients with ATN it is usually less than 1.1.

High Dose Intravenous Urogram

Even when urine volumes are extremely low, and however high the blood urea, it should be possible to obtain a characteristic appearance, providing the investigation is carefully carried out. Modern contrast media are not nephrotoxic and, although usually excreted by the kidney, are also eliminated through the biliary system.

Technique of High Dose IVU in Patients with Advanced Renal Failure

The patient should not be dehydrated prior to undergoing high dose IVU, but effective bowel preparation increases the value of the results. The examination starts with a control film of the renal areas, taken before injection of contrast medium. All subsequent films will be compared with this film. Sodium or methylglucamine diatrizoate (Urovision) 600 mg iodine/kg body weight (or 2 ml/kg) should be given by rapid intravenous injection. Further films should be taken at 5, 20 and 60 minutes and a late film at 24 hours. Tomographic cuts should be taken soon after the injection of contrast medium.

IVU Appearance in ATN

The typical IVU appearance in ATN is the development of an immediate and persistent nephrogram, which can be seen on both the 5 minute and 24 hour films. The kidneys are of normal or slightly increased size. There should be even uptake of dye throughout both kidneys, presumably due to its accumulation either in the renal tubules or in the interstitium of the renal parenchyma. No pyelogram develops. About 25 per cent of patients show a slight variation in that the nephrogram, although present at 5 minutes, becomes increasingly dense over the next 24 hours (Figure 3). Obstruction can almost always be excluded, because dilated calyces show up as negative shadows in the early films. If any doubt remains, retrograde pyelography should be performed. The demonstration of either of the two characteristic nephrographic patterns should establish the diagnosis of ATN.

However, there are some limitations to the use of high dose

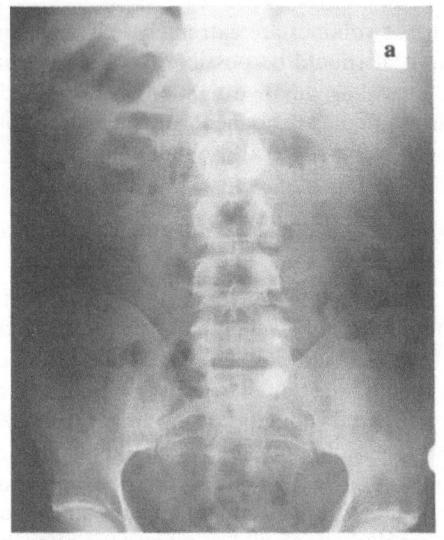

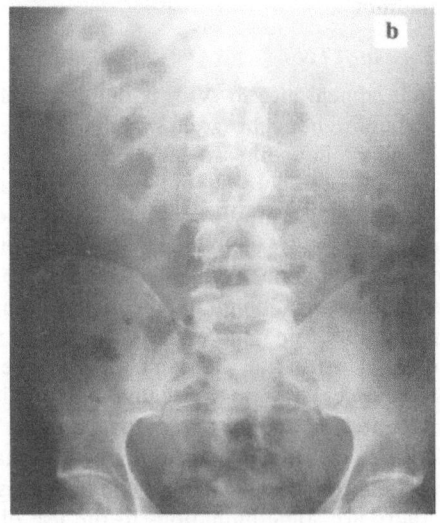

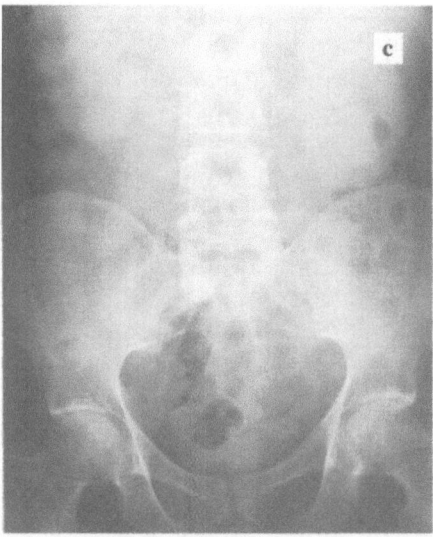

Figure 3. *High dose IVU in acute tubular necrosis. Note that the renal outline is identifiable in the preliminary films (a), but that the nephrogram is apparent in the 10 minute film (b) and very obvious in the 24 hour film (c).*

IVU. First, the patient must not be fluid overloaded, as the doses of contrast medium used contain some 100 mmol (mEq) of sodium. Second, it is impossible to transport seriously ill patients to the radiography theatre where tomography can be performed. Sometimes, however, useful information can be obtained in the ward (Figure 4).

Renal Biopsy

Renal biopsy is very rarely necessary. It is only indicated if there is real doubt about the diagnosis, particularly if glomerulonephritis is suspected because of significant proteinuria, or if the patient remains oligo/anuric for four weeks, thus raising the possibility of acute cortical necrosis. The histological appearances have been described on page 4.

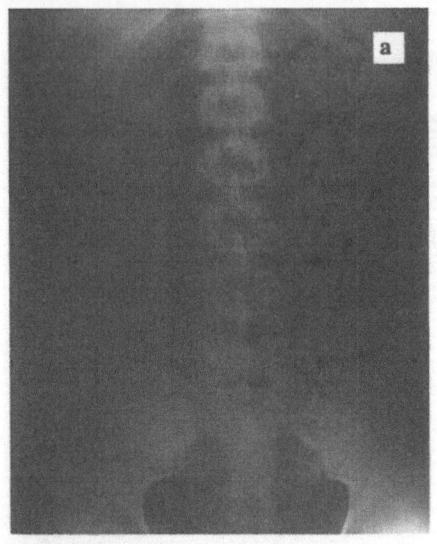

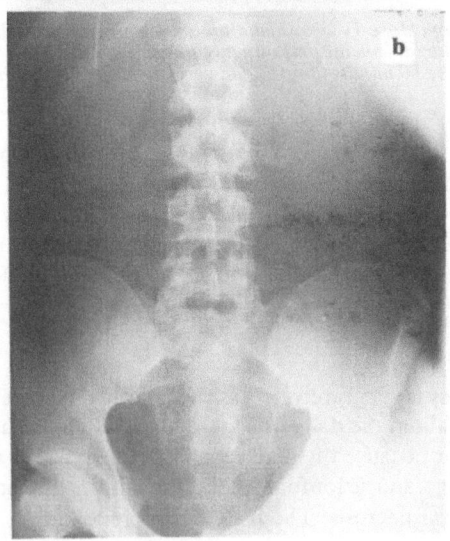

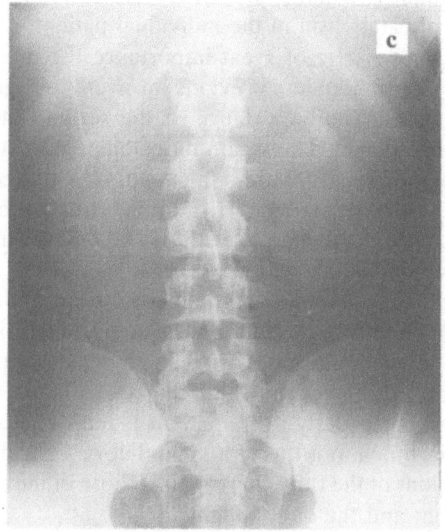

Figure 4. *IVU in acute tubular necrosis. This patient had been in a car crash and had multiple fractures and a rupture of the liver. At laparotomy an extensive retroperitoneal haematoma was seen. He remained severely oliguric and required ventilation for three weeks. The cause of his renal failure was established by a high dose IVU conducted in the intensive care unit. Although (a) the preliminary film is overexposed, (b and c) the 10 minute and 24 hour films both show a clear nephrogram. This is the most characteristic pattern seen in ATN.*

Investigations for the Management of a Patient with ATN

It is important to establish the severity of renal failure and the rate of catabolism. This can be achieved by repeated measurement of serum urea and creatinine. The urea reflects not only renal function, but also the degree of catabolism; it is raised in patients with infection, infarction, haemorrhage or tumour. Creatinine, on the other hand, reflects only renal function and lean body mass and is unchanged in catabolic states. The difference between the rate of rise of creatinine and that of urea, therefore, is a valuable guide to the degree of catabolism in the individual patient.

Electrolytes are also of great importance. Changes in serum sodium are unusual, unless previous intravenous regimens have been injudicious. The importance of the serum potassium has already been stressed. The serum bicarbonate reflects the inevitable acidosis of renal failure, which can be checked by direct measurement of the plasma pH, although this is not routinely performed. Both the degree of acidosis and the rate of rise of the serum potassium are increased in catabolic patients.

Further management requires daily monitoring of the full blood picture and platelet count, electrolytes, urea and creatinine levels. If possible, the patient should be weighed daily as this is the best guide to fluid balance. The fluid charts are liable to inherent inaccuracies, particularly if the patient is febrile, incontinent or develops diarrhoea. It is therefore mandatory to be able to check the calculations of the fluid chart against those of the clinical state of the patient and the daily weight.

Management

The treatment of the underlying condition which led to the development of ATN is often the most important part of management and need only be modified insofar as is made necessary by the lack of renal function. For example, any operation is best postponed until after the patient's uraemic state has been corrected by dialysis; it should not be cancelled.

The natural history of ATN is classically divided into the oliguric phase, the diuretic phase and the recovery of renal function.

Oliguric Phase

The oliguric phase is characterized by daily urine volumes of less than 400 ml. Some patients continue to pass larger volumes but they are exposed to many of the same risks faced by those with oliguria, and the principles of management are the same.

Hyperkalaemia

If present, hyperkalaemia is the most serious early complication of ARF and should be treated first. There are four lines of treatment but before any are instituted, the drug chart and intravenous fluid regimen should be checked to ensure that no added potassium is being given.

Intravenous calcium and sodium. The effect of potassium on the myocardial cell can be countered by intravenous calcium and sodium. Sodium is probably more effective, but has the disadvantage of adding to the dangers of fluid overload. Therefore it is usual to give 10 ml of 10 per cent calcium gluconate intravenously. This will improve the ECG almost immediately, without changing the serum potassium, but its effect is shortlived.

Glucose/insulin intravenous infusion. This combination promotes the transport of potassium into the cell and thus changes the intracellular/extracellular potassium ratio towards safety. For each unit of insulin injected between 3 and 5 g of glucose should be given. This regimen can be given either as a bolus or as a continuous infusion. It takes rather longer to act than does intravenous calcium, but its action lasts for some hours.

Chelating agents. Oral or rectal chelating agents may be used to exchange potassium for a more harmless cation. The preparation of choice is calcium resonium, because sodium resonium donates sodium ions to the patient and thus contributes to extracellular expansion and increases the danger of fluid overload. Conversely, calcium is a safe ion to give to patients with ARF, in whom the serum concentration is characteristically reduced.

Dialysis. Both peritoneal dialysis and haemodialysis can be used to remove potassium from the body, as the dialysate contains no potassium (peritoneal dialysis) or a very low concentration (1.5 mmol/l) (haemodialysis). The choice between the two methods of dialysis is discussed on page 32.

These four methods are not mutually exclusive and, indeed, in severely hyperkalaemic patients all four should be used, the effect being judged by monitoring the ECG and repeated measurements of the serum potassium. The effectiveness of these measures will depend on the degree of catabolism of the patient and thus the rate of rise in serum potassium. If the danger of hyperkalaemia is recognized, treatment is almost always effective, and hyperkalaemia has become a rare cause of death. Late diagnosis remains the main danger.

Fluid Regimens and the Place of Diuretics

The treatment of shock. Many patients with ATN present with 'shock'—a reduced cardiac output, tachycardia and hypotension. In the early stages the patient may be warm peripherally, but if corrective measures are not taken, the periphery becomes cold and clammy. Treatment is standard: adequate intravenous fluid replacement, oxygen, antibiotics if indicated, and the patient should be nursed flat or even head down. In other words, the same principle applies to the patient in renal failure as to any other shocked patient. If these measures are not successful in restoring the cardiac output, the prognosis is poor, but several regimens have been suggested.

Digoxin. This drug should be avoided in renal failure unless there are sound indications for its use, because it is largely excreted by the kidney. The best practice is to give only a digitalizing dose. Continued administration is often unnecessary as the crisis is usually resolved within 48 hours.

High dose steroids. The intravenous administration of 1 g of methyl prednisolone frequently raises blood pressure and cardiac output, but it also greatly increases the rate of catabolism of the patient. This increases the frequency with which dialysis must be performed, which may be difficult in the hypotensive patient. It also increases the patient's liability to infection and delays wound healing.

Peripheral vasodilatation and fluid replacement. An α blocker, such as thymoxamine (which is better than phenoxybenzamine because of its shorter half-life), is used to dilate peripheral arterioles and plasma is poured into the expanded circulating space, thus improving peripheral perfusion. This therapeutic approach requires considerable expertise and the likelihood of a patient surviving both it and the shock that caused it to be attempted is remote.

Dopamine. This is the current drug of first choice in the management of shock in patients with ATN because it raises both the cardiac output, by increasing myocardial contractility, and renal blood flow. It causes constriction of the peripheral blood vessels thereby increasing the blood pressure. Dopamine is given by continuous intravenous infusion of between 1 and 20 μg/kg/min, depending on the clinical response as determined by the blood pressure. It is effective in the short term, and in low doses may increase urine output significantly, but like all the methods described, it probably has little effect on the subsequent survival of the patient.

Fluid Management in the Oliguric Patient

The assessment of the state of hydration of patients has already been detailed. Severe hypovolaemia is easily identified and the fluid loss should be apparent from the history. It should be immediately and quickly replaced, so that cardiac output and therefore renal blood flow can be restored to normal as soon as possible. Monitoring the central venous pressure is useful, particularly in elderly patients in whom the danger of inducing pulmonary oedema is ever present. Once the patient's fluid balance is corrected, urine output should be assessed over the next hour, for which it may be necessary to catheterize the patient.

If oliguria persists, intravenous frusemide starting with a conservative dose of 40 mg may be given. If oliguria still persists, this dose should be followed by 500 mg given intravenously over 15 minutes. Faster rates may cause transient dizziness and deafness. In a minority of patients an increase in the urine volume will occur, although there may be only a marginal increase in glomerular filtration rate. However, the increase in urine volume is useful in itself in that it allows more effective nutrition than if oliguria had persisted. A very few patients appear to have a substantial improvement in renal function following this therapy. For these two reasons large doses of frusemide are worth a trial. One controlled trial has shown that frusemide 2 g/day shortens the oliguric phase; however, this has not been confirmed by others and has not become common practice. Some nephrologists continue to use mannitol (20 g i.v.) with similar results, but this has the danger of exacerbating fluid overload.

If the patient's urine volume fails to increase following a large dose of frusemide or mannitol, the volume of fluid replaced depends on the estimated or measured losses which should include urine, vomit, drainage from wounds, and loss from the bowel. The insensible loss through the skin and with respiration is about 1 litre/day, but 500 ml of water is made available by normal metabolism. Therefore, 500 ml/day is usually allowed for insensible loss, but this increases in the pyrexial patient by an extra 500 ml for each degree C rise in body temperature. These rough rules are a guide; the state of hydration of the patient should be checked several times each day and adjustments made.

The route by which fluid is given will depend on the clinical state of the patient. It is obviously better to give fluid orally, because intravenous and even nasogastric lines increase the risk of infection and haemorrhage. However, intravenous lines are usually necessary because of the patient's overall condition. Hyperosmolar fluids must be given through a long line, which is also useful for monitoring the CVP. The electrolyte content of the chosen regimen is only important if the patient is not being dialysed, although no extra potassium should be given unless the patient is hypokalaemic. The main concerns are not only to keep the patient correctly hydrated, but also to give adequate nutrition.

Nutrition

In the rare non-catabolic patient who can eat normally and who does not require dialysis, 40 g of protein with 2,000 calories per day are adequate, easily arranged and palatable even with quite severe fluid restriction. The main problems are set by an oliguric patient who is hypercatabolic and requires parenteral nutrition. Because oliguria restricts the volume of fluid that can be given, it is seldom possible to give adequate intravenous nutrition. The nephrologist, therefore, has to design a regimen which is as near ideal as possible for a particular patient. It should be started as soon as is practical, because the patient is usually catabolic at the time the nephrologist first sees him, and it is possible that the illness will be prolonged.

The ground rules are these:

1. Nitrogen requirement: a normal 70 kg man requires between 6 and 10 g of nitrogen/day to maintain him in positive balance. In a hypercatabolic patient this may rise to nearly 50 g/day.

2. Calorie requirement: in order to utilize the nitrogen effectively, 200 cal/g of nitrogen should be given.

3. Carbohydrate requirement: at least 30 per cent of the calories should be given as carbohydrate, to ensure sufficient generation of oxaloacetate to maintain the tricarboxylic acid cycle.

The best source of nitrogen is either a hydrolysate of casein, e.g. aminosol, which has the advantage of being cheaper, or a synthetic crystalline L-amino acid solution (e.g. Synthamin 17), as D-amino acids are not utilized. These synthetic preparations are free from peptides and ammonia. In practice, both types are equally effective in maintaining nitrogen balance. The importance of regimens containing nitrogen in improving the prognosis of the patient has been confirmed by a clinical trial, and animal experiments have shown that nitrogen administration increases the speed of recovery of renal function due to faster regeneration of tubular cells.

The best carbohydrate to give is glucose. It provides 4 cal/g, but is dependent on insulin for its metabolism. Hyperglycaemia almost inevitably develops when 50 per cent dextrose is used, because uraemic patients are relatively insulin resistant. Therefore, the blood glucose concentration must be measured regularly to assess insulin requirements.

The method of insulin administration poses problems because if it is mixed with glucose in the bottle, it adheres to the glass and most of it is lost. If it is infused separately through a constant infusion device, the patient risks hypoglycaemia when the glucose infusion is stopped, unless the insulin is discontinued at the same time. The adherence of insulin to glass can be lessened by adding a small amount of human serum albumin to the dextrose solution and this may be the method of choice. Fructose is less desirable as a source of carbohydrate because of the risk of lactic acidosis, particularly if hepatic insufficiency is also present. Sorbitol is slowly metabolized to fructose which in turn is changed to glucose. It therefore offers no advantage.

Intravenous fat is a very useful preparation because it provides 9 cal/g and because it reduces the amount of glucose required. Soya bean derivatives (Intralipid) are safer than cotton seed derivatives and remain the preparation of choice. The limitations of Intralipid are that not more than 1 litre of the 20 per cent preparation should be infused in 24 hours, and it should not be used in patients who are actively bleeding or who have severe hepatic dysfunction. The serum turbidity should also be checked some hours after the end of infusion to ensure that the fat has been metabolized; no further Intralipid should be given until the serum appears clear.

Alcohol provides about 7 cal/g but can only be used in limited quantities for obvious reasons, and has been used as such, e.g. in aminosol–fructose–ethanol.

Thus an ideal regimen for a catabolic patient requiring 30 g of nitrogen/day would consist of 2 litres of synthamin 17, 2 litres of 50 per cent dextrose and 1 litre of 20 per cent Intralipid. Unfortunately, it is seldom possible to give 5 litres to an anuric patient, and most 'hypercatabolic' patients with ATN remain in negative nitrogen balance and lose muscle mass. Repeated dialysis enables more fluid to be given and this is perhaps the most important reason for undertaking early and frequent dialysis.

The complications of parenteral feeding primarily relate to the risks of an indwelling long line. Great care should be taken to keep the puncture sites sterile and ideally the catheter should be replaced every 7 to 14 days.

It is difficult to assess the contribution of adequate parenteral nutrition to the survival of patients with ATN. One controlled study showed that dextrose/nitrogen feeding regimens were superior to dextrose alone, but no other controlled trials exist and they would now be considered unethical.

In patients undergoing dialysis it is important that water soluble vitamins be replaced. Clinically folate deficiency appears first (often as thrombocytopenia), but this may be because it is most easily recognized. It is best to start patients on folic acid and other water soluble vitamins as soon as dialysis is undertaken.

Infections

Infections are the main or contributing cause of ATN in about one-third of patients and develop in a further 50 per cent. The management and prevention of these infections is of major importance and the failure of therapy is a common cause of death. The common sites are the lung, urine and wounds; septicaemia is found in about 15 per cent of patients.

Table 7. Infections in ATN. (Modified from Zech et al., *Advances in Nephrology*, 1971.) Order of frequency of appearances in various sites.

Blood
Staphylococcus
Streptococcus
E. coli
Pseudomonas
Proteus

Lung
S. aureus
Enterococcus
Klebsiella
Pseudomonas
Proteus

Urine
Enterococcus
E. coli
Klebsiella
Proteus
Pseudomonas

Many infections are caused by organisms acquired in hospital which are frequently resistant to commonly used antibiotics (Table 7). Therefore, the choice of antibiotics should ideally depend on the result of relevant cultures and the sensitivity of the offending organism. However, the clinical condition of the patient is often so critical that immediate action is required and the choice of antibiotics remains empirical. Table 8 lists the desirable antibiotics and those that are best avoided.

Antibiotic Choice

The most commonly used antibiotic in patients with ATN is the aminoglycoside gentamicin, which is entirely excreted by the kidney. The dose must be modified and serum levels checked frequently to ensure that the dose chosen produces therapeutic levels. Nothing is more discouraging than to have a patient recover from a life-threatening illness only to find that he has permanent dizziness so disabling that he lacks the confidence even to go out of doors without support. In practice, it is comparatively easy to give gentamicin to the anuric patient receiving either peritoneal or haemodialysis, as the regimens are well understood. The same rules apply to other aminoglycosides. Lincomycin is also frequently used, particularly in patients with faecal peritonitis following bowel perforation or the breakdown of anastomoses after an operation on the bowel. It can be given in normal doses to patients with normal hepatic function. Diarrhoea is common, but

Table 8. Antibiotic choice in ATN.

Desirable	Undesirable
All penicillins	Tetracycline
Carbenicillin	Chloramphenicol
Cephalothin	Cephaloridine
Gentamicin	Nalidixic acid
Amikacin	Nitrofurantoin
Lincomycin	
Metronidazole	
Co-trimoxazole (rarely indicated)	

is not apparent in patients with an ileus! Pseudomembranous enterocolitis is much rarer, but is such a serious complication that metronidazole is used with increasing frequency. As previously discussed, antibiotics of the penicillin group can be given in normal doses; it is better to avoid the cephalosporins, but if one must be used, cephalothin is probably the drug of choice.

Nursing Care

Although antibiotics are important in the management of infection, various nursing measures should never be forgotten, and may be even more important in preventing the development of infection. For example, two-hourly mouth washes have almost eradicated parotitis, which used to be such a scourge of patients with ATN. Regular search for oral thrush is mandatory, as perhaps the most common cause of chest pain in these patients is *Candida oesophagitis*. There is little point in having a urethral catheter in situ in an anuric patient unless there has been direct trauma to the urethra, so once the diagnosis has been established, it should be removed. Correct care of intravenous cannulae dramatically reduces the incidence of infections attributable to this source. Long lines should be changed at least once a fortnight and peripheral intravenous lines more frequently.

Catabolic uraemic patients on ventilators are particularly liable to develop bed sores and their prevention is only possible by meticulous and thorough nursing care. Wounds heal slowly, so sutures should not be removed at the usual time, as they do little harm while in situ but a burst abdomen could kill the patient. They should not be removed until the oliguric phase is over or until after two weeks, whichever is the shorter.

Regular chest physiotherapy will prevent the development of basal atelectasis which is the common starting point for chest infections, particularly in patients undergoing peritoneal dialysis. It is also an important part of the management of established chest infection. For all these reasons, most patients with ATN are best managed in an intensive care area where they can be assigned a nurse each.

Disseminated Intravascular Coagulation (DIC)

The diagnosis of disseminated intravascular coagulation is made by the finding of prolongation of the prothrombin time, PTTK, or the thrombin time associated with thrombocytopenia, increased bilirubin concentration and elevated levels of fibrin degradation products; fragments of red cells are frequently seen on blood film. Not all these features may be present in each patient, but some evidence of DIC is found in about 20 per cent of patients with ATN, many of whom also have septicaemia or some other form of infection.

The presence of DIC is valuable but indirect evidence of infection, unless another obvious cause (such as a mismatched blood transfusion or amniotic fluid embolism) is apparent. Its detection no longer carries any therapeutic implications other than to undertake a diligent search for the underlying cause and to assess the efficacy of treatment in removing it. Heparin is now rarely used to prevent further consumption of the coagulation factors.

Anaemia

Anaemia is an inevitable consequence of ARF, as a result of uraemia, infection and often blood loss. It should be corrected by regular transfusion. There is an advantage in keeping the haemoglobin level as near normal as possible in patients who are critically ill and in whom pulmonary function is frequently defective.

Gastrointestinal Haemorrhage

Gastrointestinal haemorrhage occurs in about 20 per cent of patients with ATN, particularly those who have undergone abdominal surgery, suffered extensive trauma, had severe burns, or are otherwise extremely ill. Haemorrhage may start slowly, first being detected by a change of colour of the nasogastric aspirate. Endoscopic examination may show a single peptic ulcer, but a more common appearance is that of multiple shallow ulcers. Surgical treatment of haemorrhage is therefore often unsuccessful, and in any case the patient is usually not fit enough to undergo extensive surgery. Treatment relies on correcting coagulation defects and improving the metabolic environment by early and frequent dialyses. The role of cimetidine has not yet been assessed, but in view of the hypergastrinaemia found in renal failure, it could be a major advance.

Dialysis

The majority of patients who develop ATN require some form of dialysis during the oliguric period. Dialysis is capable of removing the waste products of nitrogen metabolism, including urea and creatinine, correcting acidosis and electrolyte disturbances, and removing fluid.

The indications for dialysis are relative, but it is now common practice to start dialysis earlier in the development of renal failure than in the past, in the hope that cellular function will be better maintained. For example, lymphocyte response to PHA in in vitro cultures is better when the cells are cultured in serum taken from the patient after dialysis than when the same patient's pre-dialysis serum is used. Obviously there are not many cells whose function can be tested in this way, but the generalization has been accepted. Further indirect evidence is that if the blood urea is allowed to rise above a certain level, its rate of rise accelerates, suggesting that a very uraemic environment contributes to catabolism. Therefore, the following are guidelines as to when dialysis should be started in ARF, but there may be reasons for disregarding them in an individual patient:

1. Serum urea concentration above 35 mmol/l ($\simeq$ 200 mg/dl).

2. Serum potassium value of more than 6.5 mmol/l (6.5 mEq/l).

3. Marked acidosis with a bicarbonate of below 12 mmol/l (12 mEq/l).

4. Fluid overload, particularly in the presence of pulmonary oedema.

5. A confused uncooperative patient in whom conservative management is impracticable. Although renal failure itself does not cause confusion, convulsions or abnormal neurological signs except terminally, it probably contributes to their appearance in patients who have widespread infection or inappropriate drug

therapy. However, an alternative explanation, such as a subdural haematoma, should always be excluded.

6. The development of haemorrhage, particularly from the gastrointestinal tract.

7. To ensure earlier and adequate calorie administration.

Choice of Dialysis Method

The method of dialysis chosen depends on the presentation of the patient and the unit in which he is being treated. As a general rule, haemodialysis is preferable to peritoneal dialysis because it is more efficient in correcting uraemia and is not so liable to introduce infection. However, it does require the insertion of an arteriovenous silastic shunt, which is usually placed in the forearm, using local anaesthesia. This is a small operation which can, if necessary, be performed in intensive care areas or a side room. If the possibility of chronic renal failure cannot be excluded or if the diagnosis is unknown, the shunt should be placed in the vessels at the ankle, as the forearm vessels may be subsequently required for the creation of an arteriovenous fistula for use for regular dialysis. Once the shunt has been inserted, it is ready for immediate use. Therefore it should be possible to start haemodialysis within two hours of making a decision to do so. The frequency with which the patient requires dialysis depends on his rate of catabolism: most require four to six hours dialysis on alternate days.

There are two main limitations to the efficiency of haemodialysis. First, it can be technically difficult to achieve satisfactory dialysis in hypotensive patients with a reduced cardiac output, because this causes a low flow through the artificial kidney with a subsequent reduction in efficiency. Second, haemodialysis requires that blood flowing extracorporeally be heparinized, which may exacerbate any haemorrhagic tendency of the patient. It is possible to perform regional heparinization by adding suitable doses of protamine to blood returning from the machine, but this is technically difficult. It is best simply to add as little heparin as is consistent with the prevention of clotting in the lines, controlling the dose by frequent measurements of the whole blood clotting time and aiming at values between 8 and 12 minutes.

Peritoneal dialysis is much simpler than haemodialysis and can be performed in any hospital. The peritoneal catheter can be sited under local anaesthesia in the ward within minutes of the decision to dialyse being taken. However, there are many patients in whom this procedure is unsuitable, the most frequent being those with recent abdominal surgery with drains remaining in situ. If it is known that the patient will require dialysis postoperatively, a peritoneal catheter can be placed by the surgeon at the end of the operation and the peritoneum made watertight. Leakage of peritoneal fluid either into the chest or into the abdominal wall or through wounds can complicate the patient's management and is a potential route for dissemination of infection. Although peritoneal dialysis is much less efficient than haemodialysis, its effectiveness can be increased by ensuring that the peritoneal dialysis fluid is at 37 °C at the moment it runs into the patient's abdomen, and by making sure that two or three litres of the fluid are exchanged hourly.

Even when practical, this form of dialysis has many drawbacks. It is not efficient enough to manage the 'hypercatabolic' patient; the residual volume of fluid in the peritoneum splints the diaphragm and increases the chance of chest infection; peritonitis is a common complication; mechanical failures, particularly difficulties with draining fluid out of the peritoneum, are frequent; and up to 60 g of protein are lost in the effluent each 24 hours, which adds to the problem of providing adequate nutrition. However, its simplicity makes it the method of choice in some patients, particularly those presenting with 'medical' causes of ATN in whom catabolism is rarely extreme. Its other great advantage is that it permits more regular fluid removal and thus allows a more liberal fluid regimen.

Subsequent Visits to the Patient

The nephrologist has to assess repeatedly the effect of therapy on the patient and balance the various risks and benefits of any particular treatment appropriate to the primary condition but potentially damaging to renal recovery. But although his job is to think for the kidneys, the priority remains the effective treatment of the underlying condition, because renal recovery almost always occurs providing that the patient survives.

Diuretic Phase

The oliguric phase lasts on average about 10 days, although this may vary between one and 40 days and even longer periods have been reported. It gradually merges into the diuretic phase as urine volumes increase at first undramatically but then doubling up daily. Urine volumes of more than 3 litres/day are rare in a patient who has remained in correct fluid balance, but even with this volume the GFR remains very low and, therefore, dialysis may have to be continued well into the diuretic phase. However, sodium and potassium losses rise substantially, and the replacement of these cations is important; in particular, potassium has to be added to the dialysate to prevent significant depletion.

The patient's general condition often improves dramatically during this phase; infections clear up, the patient can be weaned off the ventilator, bowel sounds return and oral feeding can often be started.

Table 9. Prognosis in ATN (subgroup % mortality).

Author	Period	Medical	Surgical	Traumatic	Obstetric	Total
Kleinknecht	1968*	55	54	55	15	42
Kleinknecht	1971*	37	38	33	8	29
Kennedy	1959–1970	36	61	50	21	44
Stott	1969–1971	—	65	—	20	57
Hall	1955–1967	64	47	72	21	53

* Comparison to show benefit of early haemodialysis.
Kleinknecht, D. et al., *Advances in Nephrology*, 1971, **1**, 207.
Kennedy, A. C. et al., *Quart. J. Med.*, 1973, **42**, 73.
Stott, R. B. et al., *Lancet*, 1972, **2**, 75.
Hall, J. N. et al., 1970, *Ann. intern. Med.*, **73**, 515.

Recovery of Renal Function

As the diuretic phase continues, renal function gradually returns. This can present problems in adjusting the dose of drugs excreted by the kidney, because doses have to be changed regularly to maintain effective levels. It is often possible to stop giving drugs, but if not, the dose given should be guided by measuring the serum concentration. Complete recovery of renal function does occur, although the GFR of many patients is permanently reduced by up to 60 per cent. The ability to acidify and concentrate the urine gradually returns to near normal, so the patient has no long-term serious renal sequelae of the episode of ATN.

Statistics of ATN

A very real disappointment has been the failure over the last 10 to 15 years to improve significantly the prognosis of patients presenting with ATN. The introduction of parenteral nutrition and the use of early dialysis have been shown to improve survival, and yet half the patients continue to die. The most frequent cause of death (about 70 per cent) remains the precipitating illness and only 10 per cent die as a result of renal failure, e.g. hyperkalaemia. However, most patients die with uncontrolled infection, and uraemia depresses almost all defensive mechanisms which, although improved by adequate nutrition and frequent dialysis, apparently remain incapable of eradicating advanced infection. (Whether a non-uraemic patient would be capable of doing so is unknown.) There is unlikely to be any improvement in the survival of patients with ARF until a new approach to the management of their infections has been developed.

The mortality associated with the main clinical subgroups of patients described in various series is shown in Table 9. It can be seen that patients presenting with an obstetric cause of ATN almost always survive, whereas the mortality of surgical cases is several times higher. Groups of patients with a particularly bad or good prognosis are listed in Table 10.

Table 10. ATN prognosis.

Very poor prognosis

Extensive burns

By-pass surgery

Sepsis following abdominal surgery

Trauma to abdomen and thorax

Severe hepatic failure

Paraquat poisoning

Criminal abortion associated with clostridial infection

Any patient requiring ventilation for more than 48 hours

Good prognosis

Obstetrical accidents without sepsis

Mismatched blood transfusions

Trauma to limbs

Viral infection (e.g. coxsackie, influenza) causing myoglobinuria

Some nephrotoxins

References

Sharpstone, P., Prescribing for patients with renal failure, *Br. Med. J.*, 1977, **2**, 36.

3. Cortical Necrosis

The term cortical necrosis describes bilateral massive necrosis of both glomeruli and tubules, causing permanent loss of renal function. It is probably caused by the same mechanisms as those causing ATN; therefore the degree of recovery depends on how much of the cortex has been affected. Presumably a degree of cortical necrosis is common, and this explains the permanent reduction in GFR found in many patients after an episode of ATN. However, the full blown syndrome in which there is no recovery of renal function is very rare. The diagnosis is usually suspected when oliguria persists for more than four weeks, but there are clinical clues which may raise suspicions earlier. It is much commoner in accidents of pregnancy which account for 50 per cent of patients described. Heavy proteinuria or total anuria (both rare in patients with ATN) may also arouse suspicion.

Investigations

If the patient remains severely oliguric after four weeks, further investigations are indicated. A plain abdominal radiograph may show cortical calcification as early as four weeks; this subsequently extends into a characteristic tramline around the kidney. Renal arteriography may demonstrate patchy normal areas surrounded by shrunken avascular cortex and filling of the subcapsular vessels. Renal biopsy is diagnostic when it shows changes of cortical infarction, but it is possible to take the biopsy sample from a small area of relatively normal tissue.

Management

The management of the patient is similar to that in ATN until recovery from the precipitating illness occurs. Thereafter, the patient should be assessed for regular dialysis which, if appropriate, should be instituted as soon as possible. Accelerated hypertension is a late complication which may necessitate bilateral nephrectomy.

4. The Hepatorenal Syndrome

Although the name of this syndrome is known widely, the disorder which it describes is not well defined. There are four basic associations between the two organs which might come under this heading.

1. Reduced cardiac output giving rise to ATN and hepatocellular dysfunction. Hepatic function is usually maintained in most patients with ATN. Jaundice due to hepatocellular necrosis is an ominous sign, and is most commonly seen in those who develop ATN following open heart surgery. The patient is frequently on a ventilator, requiring little sedation, and small areas of petechial haemorrhage can be found. Such patients rarely survive.

2. Drugs or toxins causing ATN and hepatocellular necrosis. There are numerous chemicals that are known to do this, of which paracetamol, ethyleneglycol and carbon tetrachloride are the most common (Plate 3).

3. The increased postoperative incidence of ATN following operations for the relief of biliary obstruction. Dawson (1968) showed that patients undergoing simple surgical procedures for the relief of obstruction were liable to develop renal failure and the severity of the jaundice was proportional to the risk of renal failure. He showed that all patients undergoing surgery had a fall in the creatinine clearance, which was most marked in jaundiced patients and was proportional to bilirubin levels. It could be ameliorated by infusing 500 ml of 10 per cent mannitol beginning two hours before surgery and sufficient five per cent mannitol postoperatively to maintain a urine flow of 1 ml/min over the next

24 hours. This practice has reduced the incidence of ATN in jaundiced patients.

4. Oliguric renal failure associated with advanced liver disease, particularly cirrhosis. This is the association to which the term hepatorenal syndrome was originally applied. Most patients with terminal hepatic failure die of renal insufficiency. The urinary sodium is characteristically low and is associated with hyponatraemia. The cause is not clear, but renal blood flow is dramatically reduced despite a slightly increased cardiac output. Renal function only returns if there is spontaneous improvement of the liver disorder.

References

Dawson, J. L., Acute postoperative renal failure in obstructive jaundice, *Ann. R. Coll. Surg. Engl.*, 1968, **42,** 163.

5. Structural Changes of Renal Vasculature and Glomerulonephritis Causing Renal Failure

Lesions of the Main Renal Arteries

Lesions of the main renal arteries are a very rare cause of acute renal failure, but have been described in three situations.

Trauma

Severe trauma can cause rupture of the renal artery, either by direct damage to the intima of the artery with subsequent occlusion, or by avulsion as the result of violent deceleration. These injuries are usually fatal, but survival has been reported. An IVU will show an absent nephrogram, and arteriography shows tapering of the main renal artery. Surgical repair should be attempted if the patient's condition justifies the risk.

Renal Artery Embolus

Renal artery embolus is quite a common event, but seldom leads to renal failure. The patient complains of loin pain and may have frank haematuria. It is associated with the same radiological changes as those of direct trauma to the renal artery. Embolectomy may be successful even after a delay of 12 hours.

Dissection of Abdominal Aortic Aneurysm Involving Both Renal Arteries

Dissection of an abdominal aortic aneurysm is again rare, but surgical replacement of an abdominal aortic aneurysm by a prosthesis commonly leads to renal failure. This is usually due to ATN unless the renal arteries are involved, in which case infarction may result and recovery is unusual.

Lesions of the Renal Microvasculature

Accelerated Hypertension

Hypertension usually causes renal failure to develop insidiously, but occasionally patients with accelerated hypertension present with acute renal failure. The unfortunate patient often has a forceful left ventricular impulse and a loud aortic second sound. Papilloedema with exudates and haemorrhages is almost always present, and areas of purpura are sometimes found. The blood film reveals fragmented red cells and thrombocytopenia, although the coagulation screen may be nearly normal. Proteinuria (if urine is produced) is usual. An IVU performed as described above produces a very poor nephrogram, but the kidneys are smooth and of normal size. Renal biopsy can be performed once the blood pressure has been controlled and the platelet count has risen above $100 \times 10^9/l$. On biopsy, the glomeruli appear avascular with crinkling of the glomerular basement membrane. Arterioles show intimal proliferation with virtual occlusion of the lumen and fibrinoid material is present within the walls of some arteries and arterioles.

Treatment

Treatment involves radical control of hypertension aiming to keep the diastolic pressure below 95 mm Hg. Dialysis should be used to remove fluid and to control uraemia. Within two to four weeks there should be improvement in the fundal appearances, but return of some renal function is rare, perhaps occurring in only 10 per cent of patients. However, regular dialysis treatment with transplantation is often successful, although bilateral nephrectomy may be necessary to control the hypertension.

Haemolytic Uraemic Syndrome

Haemolytic uraemic syndrome (HUS) is a rare disease of unknown aetiology affecting children mainly below the age of 2 years of either sex. It usually occurs sporadically but small epidemics have been reported. It frequently presents with diarrhoea and fever lasting a few days, followed by acute renal failure, haemolytic anaemia and thrombocytopenia. The child becomes ill and irritable and focal neurological signs may appear. Hypertension may be absent at the onset but develops later. The prognosis is variable, being worse in older children. About 20 per cent die in the acute stage and a further 20 per cent progress more slowly to renal failure. Some have permanent neurological sequelae. Complete recovery occurs in 25 per cent and the remainder survive with a permanent reduction in renal function.

Diagnosis is based on the clinical presentation and the demonstration of microangiopathic haemolytic anaemia on the blood film (fragmented red cells, microspherocytes and helmet cells) associated with thrombocytopenia and renal failure. Renal biopsy is only possible when the bleeding disorder has been corrected. The main abnormality is in the arteries and arterioles which show necrosis, thrombosis and fibrin deposition. The glomeruli may be shrunken with areas of necrosis.

Treatment

Treatment centres on the management of renal failure and control of hypertension which frequently develops. Steroids and heparin have both been used extensively, but their efficacy remains unproven.

Thrombotic Thrombocytopenic Purpura (Moschowitz's Syndrome)

Moschowitz's syndrome is very similar to the haemolytic–uraemic syndrome, but it occurs in adults. The aetiology is also unknown, and the condition is even rarer than HUS. Clinically it comprises fever, signs of cerebral irritability, haemolytic anaemia, purpura due to increased platelet consumption and renal failure. The pathological changes in the blood and kidneys are similar to those described in HUS. The prognosis is bad, as few survivors have been described.

Treatment with large doses of steroids and heparin is usually given on an empirical basis, and recently recovery has been reported after exchange of large volumes of the patient's plasma with normal plasma.

Postpartum Nephrosclerosis

Postpartum nephrosclerosis was first described in 1968. It is very rare. As its name implies, it follows pregnancy (which has usually been quite normal) by an interval of two to 12 weeks. Renal failure and haemolytic anaemia develop insidiously. Recovery is unusual, and steroids and heparin therapy are usually given. The disease appears to be self-limiting, the patient being left with severe renal failure and hypertension. Therefore regular dialysis treatment can be successful, although nephrectomy may be required to control hypertension.

Glomerulonephritis

Both acute exudative (or post-streptococcal) glomerulonephritis and rapidly progressive (or crescentic) glomerulonephritis are associated with ARF. The kidney may be the only organ involved, or it may be part of a more generalized illness such as occurs in systemic lupus erythematosus, polyarteritis nodosa, Wegener's granulomatosis, Henoch–Schönlein purpura or Goodpasture's syndrome. Early diagnosis is essential and rests on the clinical history, presence of proteinuria and cellular casts, and the demonstration of a poor nephrogram on IVU. Both kidneys are either normal in size or enlarged; renal biopsy should be performed as soon as possible. A full description of these syndromes appears in another title in this series: *Renal Glomerular Diseases* (Sharpstone 1980).

Renal Vein Thrombosis

Renal vein thrombosis is most commonly seen in infants who become dehydrated as a result of diarrhoea and vomiting; those born of diabetic mothers are particularly vulnerable. Renal vein thrombosis causes acute loin pain and large tender kidneys. One or both kidneys may be affected, but renal failure may develop even with unilateral disease. Recovery has been described after unilateral nephrectomy, which should be considered if severe coagulation defects are present. It is often followed by an improvement in the infant's general condition and a return of renal function. However, recovery also occurs with conservative measures including rehydration and anticoagulants, and this is the method of management most frequently employed.

Renal vein thrombosis rarely occurs in adults unless the kidney itself is abnormal. Classically it is associated with amyloid, membranous nephropathy or a transplanted kidney. Diagnosis is made by renal venography which can be difficult to interpret. Its effect on renal function is variable. Thrombectomy is occasionally successful, but should only be attempted if there has been a sudden and recent reduction in renal function. Anticoagulants have also been used, but since the natural history of the syndrome is unknown it is difficult to evaluate their effectiveness.

6. Obstruction of the Renal Tract

Obstruction leads to acute renal failure only when both kidneys are involved. However, about one person in 2,000 has a solitary kidney, therefore unilateral obstruction can cause renal failure. It is also possible that infection may occur above the obstruction and cause septicaemia and ATN of the other non-obstructed kidney. More commonly, one kidney becomes obstructed silently, and only when the other renal tract becomes involved does renal failure supervene. Any obstruction of the urethra leads to bilateral involvement, but usually presents with chronic renal insufficiency.

Aetiology

The likeliest cause of obstruction varies with the age of the patient. Thus, in the first decade of life, congenital abnormalities are the most common, but in men over 65 years prostatic hypertrophy and carcinoma of the bladder, and in women over 60 years carcinoma of the uterus are the commonest causes.

Clinical Features

Acute obstructive uropathy usually presents with anuria, but rapidly advancing renal failure in the presence of a continued urine output and even polyuria does occur. Loin pain on the affected side is frequent and classical renal colic is an obvious clue. However, many patients may report no more than a slight discomfort. Urethral obstruction leads to painful distension of the bladder. Stasis of the urine predisposes to infection, which may dominate the clinical presentation.

On examination, one or both kidneys may be tender or the bladder palpable. The external meatus should always be inspected for stenosis. Pelvic examination may lead to a diagnosis of intrapelvic malignancy or prostatic hypertrophy. Patients tend to be fluid overloaded and modest hypertension is commonly seen. Sometimes ascites may be detected, but this does not always indicate malignancy.

Investigations

The degree of renal failure and the serum potassium level should be determined quickly. A high dose IVU with a 24 hour film and tomography should be obtained as an emergency. The characteristic appearance is of an enlarged kidney(s); in the early films there are large negative calyceal shadows with surrounding cortex showing the nephrographic blush. In the later films, the dye is concentrated in large distended calyces and in the pelvis. Sometimes a dilated ureter can be discerned, but it is difficult to ascertain at which level the obstruction is sited, because dye may not permeate into the stagnant urine above the obstruction.

If obstruction is demonstrated, or if it cannot be excluded with certainty, retrograde pyelograms should be performed. If it is possible to pass a catheter above the obstruction, it should be left in place. Some patients are not fit to undergo retrograde catheterization, which may entail a general anaesthetic, or they may be unsuitable, because their ureters have been implanted into a loop of bowel; in these rare patients antegrade pyelography should be performed. It is very easy to pass a lumbar puncture needle from the back into a dilated calyx and inject dye into the calyceal system. If obstruction is confirmed, a drainage catheter can be inserted and left in situ.

Treatment
Relief of Obstruction

Temporary relief can be obtained by leaving a retrograde or antegrade catheter in situ. Despite their narrow lumina, effective drainage of the kidney can be obtained. However, neither is satisfactory, as they rarely remain in the correct position. This time should be used to prepare the patient for surgical relief.

Relief of Uraemia

The patient may be unfit for surgical procedures and may require dialysis to correct uraemia. Peritoneal dialysis is usually appropriate and, if malignant obstruction is considered, the first peritoneal effluent fluid should be sent for cytological examination.

Postobstruction Diuresis

Following relief of acute obstruction, a diuresis of several litres may occur in the first 24 hours. Sodium and potassium losses are large. Therefore, an intravenous infusion should be set up at the time of the operation and accurate hourly fluid charts kept. The urinary sodium and potassium concentration should be measured, and an appropriate replacement regimen prescribed. Frequent checks of the serum electrolytes should be made. The diuresis usually lasts about three days, and care should be taken not to continue to replace unnecessarily large volumes of fluid, thus contributing to the maintenance of the diuresis. The degree of recovery of renal function depends on the severity of the obstruction and the length of time it has been in existence. Animal studies suggest that if the ureter is tied off for seven days or more, permanent reduction in GFR follows release of the obstruction. Studies in man are difficult to interpret, but the safe clinical rule is that urinary obstructions should be treated as an emergency, thus preserving as much renal function as possible.

Further Reading

Cattell, W. R., Acute renal failure. In: *Recent Advances in Renal Disease.* Jones, N. F. (Ed.) Edinburgh: Churchill Livingstone, 1975, Ch. 1, 1–47.

Kennedy, A. C., Burton, J. A., Luke, R. G. *et al.,* Factors affecting the prognosis of acute renal failures. *Q. J. Med.,* 1973, **42**: 73.

Kleinkrecht, D., Factors influencing immediate prognosis in acute renal failure with special reference to prophylactic haemodialysis. In: *Advances in Nephrology.* London: Year Book Medical Publishers, 1971, 1: 207–30.

Levinsky, N. G. and Alexander, E. A., Acute renal failure. In: *The Kidney.* Brenner, B. M. and Rector, F. C. (Eds.) London, Philadelphia: W. B. Saunders Co., 1976, Ch. 21, 806–37.

Chronic Renal Failure
7. Introduction

The advent of dialysis and renal transplantation has greatly increased the importance of renal failure, which is a comparatively rare disorder, affecting perhaps 120 per million of the population each year. Management of these patients has assumed social, political and even legal aspects, as well as the more common medical and psychological ones. It has also accelerated the trend towards specialization within our major hospitals and encouraged research into a great variety of problems to the benefit of numerous patients with normal renal function. The metabolism of vitamin D, the detection and epidemiology of serum hepatitis, the management of hypertension and certain types of poisoning, and the elucidation of various immunological mechanisms of cell injury are a few examples of clinical subjects advanced by the study of patients with renal failure. Indeed, it could be claimed that these few patients have provided one of the major clinical stimuli to medicine over the last decade.

Functions of the Kidney

The kidney has several functions: it eliminates the waste products of protein metabolism, excess hydrogen ions and several other toxic substances including many drugs; it has a crucial role in maintaining the volume of body fluids and their sodium and potassium content; it is also a major endocrine organ producing renin, 1,25-dihydroxycholecalciferol and erythropoietin; and several other hormones are metabolized within the kidney, of which the decrease of insulin, parathyroid hormone and perhaps gastrin catabolism, which occur in renal failure, may have clinical significance. Therefore loss of renal function may be expected to affect every cell in the body, and it is perhaps surprising that patients with advanced renal failure remain as well as they do.

Intact Nephron Hypothesis

To understand why this is so, it is important to investigate the manner in which renal function is lost. Theoretically it is possible that the power of acidification might be lost first, in which case the consequences of metabolic acidosis would dominate the clinical picture. Similarly if the kidney lost its ability to conserve potassium, the patient would die of hypokalaemia at a stage when the glomerular filtration remained relatively normal.

The classical experiments performed by Bricker and his associates led to the 'intact nephron hypothesis'. This postulates that the diseased kidney loses nephrons as units, i.e. both filtration and tubular functions are lost simultaneously. The remaining nephrons hypertrophy to cope with the increased load, and are capable of adapting their function to do so. The patient remains well until so many nephrons are lost that hypertrophy of the remainder no longer maintains the GFR, which then progressively declines. As further nephrons are lost the remainder are unable to acidify, concentrate or dilute the urine normally and the patient develops acidosis and a urine of fixed concentration. However, even at this stage, the function of the surviving tubules remains evident in some important aspects. Thus the sodium concentration in the blood remains constant, maintained by the remaining tubules decreasing the proportion of filtered sodium reabsorbed from 99 per cent to 95 per cent. Hyperkalaemia is also a late complication of chronic renal failure (CRF). The intact nephron hypothesis is generally valid and has provided a useful model.

However, some patients do appear to lose one function first, particularly when the tubules are predominantly involved in the disease process as happens with analgesic nephropathy or renal tubular acidosis. These patients may develop a sodium losing state or marked acidosis while the GFR is well maintained. The effect of renal failure on the endocrine function of the kidney also has important consequences for the patient and contributes largely to anaemia, renal osteodystrophy and hypertension, which are discussed later.

Therefore the reason why patients remain so well, even in advanced uraemia, is the orderly retreat which the kidney conducts in the face of the disease process. It has a vast reserve of function, enabling the patient to remain symptomless until 80 or 90 per cent of nephrons have been destroyed.

8. Causes

The causes of CRF are summarized in Table 11. Any series showing the relative incidence of the various causes of CRF must be viewed with some scepticism, because about one third of patients present for the first time with renal failure so advanced that even detailed investigation cannot reveal its cause. Thus, if a high dose IVU is performed and scars are present in the kidney, a diagnosis of chronic pyelonephritis is made, but if the outline is smooth and the patient has proteinuria, then chronic glomerulonephritis is the chosen diagnosis. Since there is no possibility of making a more accurate assessment and since it is usual for common things to occur commonly, a common diagnosis is chosen, thus fulfilling the axiom. Table 12 is taken from the European data summarized by Wing (1977).

Chronic Glomerulonephritis

Chronic glomerulonephritis should not be regarded as a single disease. It is a useful label and signifies that such a patient is more likely to have proteinuria, oedema and hypertension (see two other titles in this Topic Pack: Sharpstone, 1980, and Walls, 1980).

Chronic Pyelonephritis

The term chronic pyelonephritis is used to describe a radiological appearance on the IVU, namely a cortical scar with deformity of the underlying calyx or calyces. The disease process certainly starts before the age of five years and is often slowly progressive.

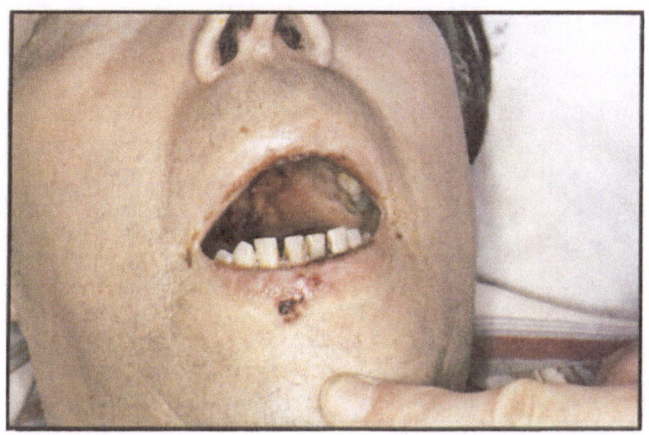

Plate 1. *Many patients with acute renal failure have dry mouths, with splitting of mucosa and secondary infection. Regular oral toilet is essential.*

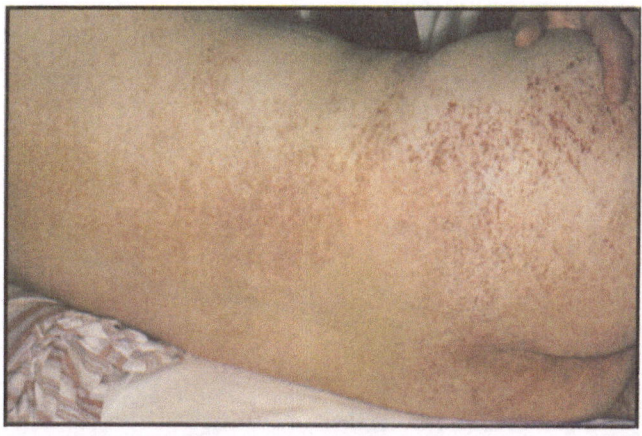

Plate 2. *Acute renal failure and diffuse petechiae. This patient had a meningococcal septicaemia.*

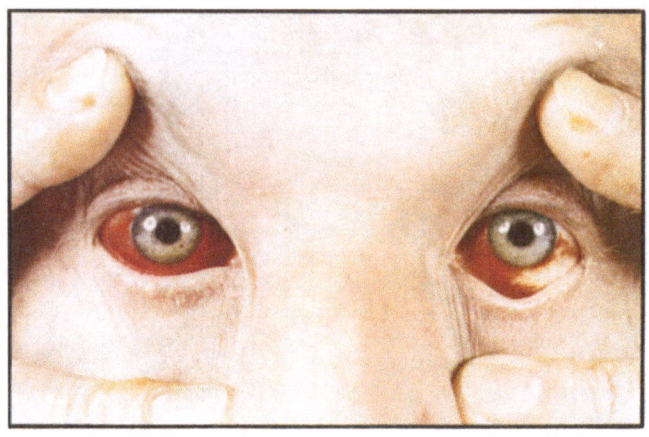

Plate 3. *Acute renal failure. There are many associations between jaundice and acute renal failure. This patient had taken an overdose of paracetamol.*

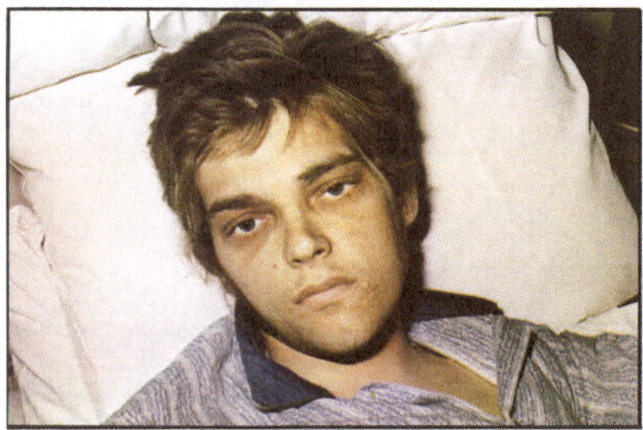

Plate 4. *Chronic renal failure. Typical skin colouring.*

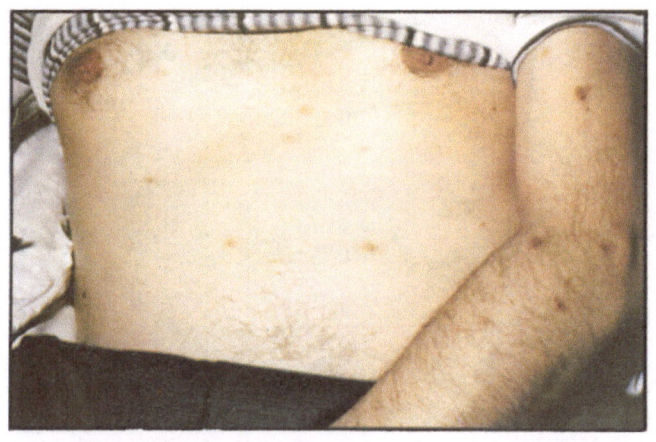

Plate 5. *Itching is common in chronic renal failure and scratching never quite relieves it although it may cause extensive damage to the skin.*

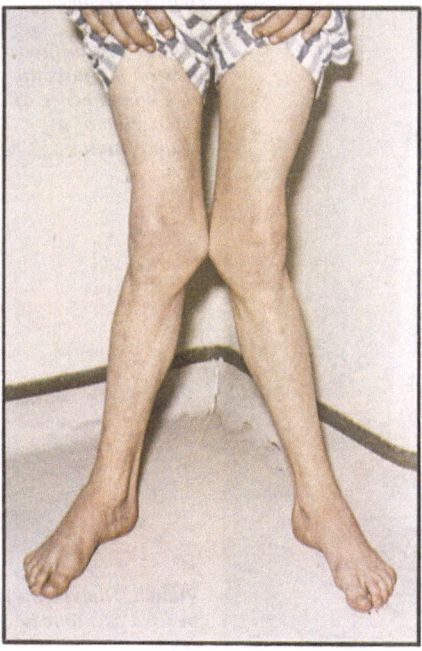

Plate 6. *Chronic renal failure. This patient had to give up football because of the deformity. He had played for a Celtic Junior Team until eight weeks before the photograph was taken.*

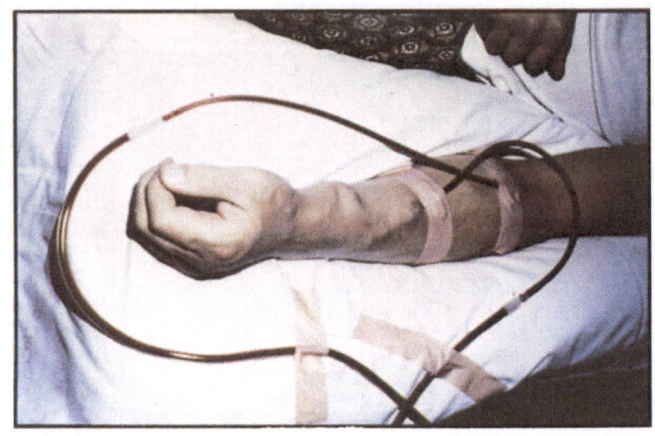

Plate 7. *Needles in position during dialysis. The tortuous veins on the forearm are a consequence of the creation of a Cimino fistula.*

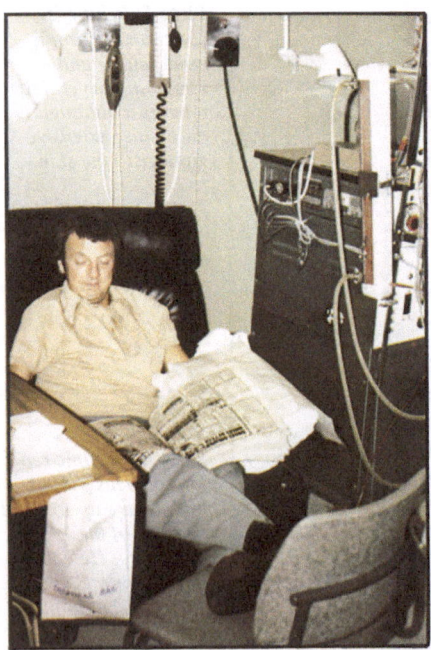

Plate 8. *Dialysis may be used as a time to relax.*

Table 11. Causes of chronic renal failure.

Glomerulonephritis
'Idiopathic'
As part of systemic disease

Chronic pyelonephritis

Chronic interstitial nephritis
Analgesia
Heavy metal
Radiation
Inherited nephritides, e.g. Alports
Balkan nephropathy

Hypertension and other vascular causes

Congenital abnormalities of the kidneys
Polycystic kidneys
Alpert's syndrome
Hypoplastic kidneys
Medullary cystic disease or nephrophthisis

Obstruction
Congenital abnormalities
Stones
Tumours
Retroperitoneal fibrosis
Prostatic hypertrophy
Urethral strictures

Metabolic diseases
Diabetes
Amyloid
Gout
Oxalosis
Hypercalcaemia and hypercalciuria

Infections
Tuberculosis
Schistosomiasis
Malaria ⎫
Infective endocarditis ⎬ Mediated by immune complexes
Chronic infections ⎭

Collagen disease
Lupus nephritis
Polyarteritis nodosa
Henoch–Schönlein purpura
Systemic sclerosis

Neurogenic bladder

Table 12. Common diagnoses made in chronic renal failure (Wing 1977).

Diagnosis	% patients
Glomerulonephritis	46.6
Glomerulonephritis (histologically examined)	(10.0)
Pyelonephritis	19.9
Drug-induced/analgesic abuse	3.3
Cystic renal disease	8.4
Hereditary/congenital	3.2
Renal vascular disease	5.4
Other identified rare diseases	9.7
Aetiology uncertain	3.5
Total no (%) of patients	47741 (100%)

Patients are more likely to suffer intermittent urinary tract infection, have a tendency to lose sodium, and hypertension is less common and less severe than in patients with glomerulonephritis. There is a higher incidence of renal osteodystrophy, perhaps because the natural history of the disease is more prolonged and these patients are often uraemic during puberty (see two other titles in this Topic Pack: Sharpstone, 1980, and Walls, 1980).

Table 13. Presenting symptoms of polycystic renal disease.

Abdominal masses
Hypertension
Urinary tract infection
Haematuria
Pain
Chronic renal failure

Polycystic Renal Disease

Polycystic renal disease is inherited as an autosomal dominant, although 30 per cent of patients have no apparent family history. It is a slowly progressive disease commonly causing terminal renal failure in the fourth and fifth decades and may present in a variety of ways (Table 13).

There are some more favourable features of renal failure due to polycystic renal disease. Anaemia is not as marked as in other forms; hypertension, although common, is generally mild and easily controlled; and a significant recovery of renal function can occur even at a late stage after correction of reversible factors. In fact, many patients remain remarkably well for months after just one short period of peritoneal dialysis. Polycystic kidneys are associated with berry aneurysms, and these patients suffer an increased incidence of subarachnoid haemorrhage. Polycystic abnormalities are also present in the lung, liver and pancreas, but are of little clinical importance.

Hypertension

Hypertension is both a common result and a frequent cause of renal failure. The development of ARF as the result of malignant hypertension has been described. Less severe, but sustained, hypertension is a cause of CRF, which has been shown to be avoidable by adequate treatment.

Obstruction

Obstruction may develop insidiously when it is not associated with oliguria. Indeed, many patients continue to pass large volumes of urine and have no symptoms, such as pain, which may alert the clinician to the underlying pathology. The causes are listed in Table 11, and diagnosis is made by high dose IVU and retrograde pyelogram. Retroperitoneal fibrosis is associated with an obstructive pattern on IVU, but no obstruction to the passage of retrograde catheters.

Analgesic Nephropathy

Analgesic nephropathy is a particularly common cause of renal failure in some countries, such as Australia and the Netherlands, but seems to be rarer in the USA. The incidence in the UK as a whole is relatively low, but is higher in Scotland than in England. Women are affected more commonly than men. One third of patients take analgesics for rheumatic complaints, another third for headaches, and the remainder consume large quantities because advertisements tell them it will make them feel better and they believe there is room for some improvement in their health. Almost all patients take compound tablets or powders containing phenacetin, of which 1 kg has usually been consumed by the time of presentation. Isolated patients have been reported who have apparently taken either aspirin or paracetamol only, but their history may be unreliable. Patients present with hypertension, haematuria, recurrent urinary tract obstruction, the passage of

Table 14. Treatable causes of CRF.

Obstructive nephropathy

Urate nephropathy

Disorders of calcium metabolism
Hyperparathyroidism
Vitamin D intoxication
Sarcoidosis
Myeloma

Collagen diseases
Lupus nephritis
Polyarteritis nodosa
Henoch–Schönlein purpura

Chronic infections
Tuberculosis
Infective endocarditis

Analgesic nephropathy

Heavy metal poisoning
Lead
Cadmium

---

papillae or chronic renal failure. Sometimes obstruction occurs if a necrotic papilla becomes detached and lodges in the ureter. Anaemia and dyspepsia are often present. If the patient can be persuaded to stop taking analgesics, renal function may improve and usually does not deteriorate further. However, about 50 per cent continue to take analgesics and progress to renal failure.

It is not yet clear whether legislation restricting the availability of phenacetin has reduced the incidence.

Other rare but correctable causes of CRF are listed in Table 14.

References

Wing, A. J., Prospects for the treatment of renal diseases. *Br. Med. J.*, 1972, **2**, 881.

9. Clinical Features

The ability of the kidney to reorganize its huge reserve of function means that patients may remain symptomless until the disease is eroding the last 10 per cent of function. Sometimes, patients present with an intermittent illness which seems unduly severe and renal failure may be detected. Some patients develop the complications of renal failure and present with bone pain or hypertension. However, the earliest symptom is usually nocturia. The total urine volume may be increased and this may be associated with thirst. The next symptom to develop is malaise, which often coincides with the development of anaemia. Exercise tolerance is reduced, but remains remarkably good even when the haemoglobin has fallen to 8 or 9 g/dl. In advanced renal failure almost every organ of the body may be affected, and it is useful to consider each separately. However, any one patient may have few of these complications or develop terminal renal failure with no other symptoms than those already described.

Cardiovascular System

Hypertension develops in about 80 per cent of patients with advanced renal failure, and its absence may indicate hypovolaemia or salt wasting. There are two main causes. Most patients have an expanded extracellular fluid volume with an increased total body sodium. Normally this would suppress the production of renin and hence angiotensin, but the concentration of both these hormones is often inappropriately raised and this combination is a potent cause of hypertension. Hypertension frequently dominates the clinical picture, causing cardiomegaly and heart failure, accelerating the rate of decline in renal function and increasing the probability of a vascular incident. Adequate control is vital and sometimes very difficult to achieve.

Atheroma, particularly of the coronary circulation, is more common in patients with renal failure and occurs at a younger age than in the normal population. Its significance is enhanced by coincidental anaemia, so that angina, myocardial infarction and peripheral vascular disease are all more common than in the normal population. Hypertensive and lipid abnormalities (types 2 and 4 hyperlipoproteinaemias) are the most obvious risk factors, but hyperuricaemia, carbohydrate intolerance and vascular calcification may be contributing factors.

Pericarditis develops in about half the patients who have terminal uraemia, but it is symptomatic in only a proportion of them. It may present as chest pain, which is eased by sitting forward, and aggravated by breathing or coughing. A pericardial friction rub is readily heard, but ECG changes are rarely typical, and echocardiography is now the investigation of choice. The detection of pericarditis is an indication for dialysis because it may herald the development of a sanguineous pericardial effusion, which may be large enough to cause cardiac tamponade.

An aortic diastolic murmur may be heard in some patients with advanced renal failure, but it disappears after a period of dialysis. The cause and significance of this are not understood.

The Skin

Uraemic patients have a characteristic pale yellow–brown colour, particularly if the course of renal failure has been protracted (Plate 4). They have a tendency to bruise easily and small intra-dermal deposits of calcium phosphate are sometimes visible. Itching is common, and in a few patients may be quite intolerable leading to persistent scratching and excoriation of all accessible areas (Plate 5). The cause for this is unknown but it has been related to underlying secondary hyperparathyroidism or to a high blood calcium × phosphate product. The classical urea frost is rarely seen since the advent of low protein diets.

Gastrointestinal Tract

Most patients develop anorexia and nausea at some time during the course of renal failure and it is usually sufficiently severe to cause some weight loss. Intermittent vomiting, particularly in the morning, is also common and it may become persistent and be associated with diarrhoea. In advanced uraemia, the diarrhoea may become blood stained, which usually signifies the development of shallow multiple ulcers of the bowel. A characteristic ammoniacal foetor is associated with advanced renal failure, and some patients complain of a distinct metallic taste which contributes towards their anorexia. The cause of many of these gastrointestinal symptoms may be a high concentration of ammonia derived from the metabolism of urea by bowel bacteria. Whatever the explanation, gastrointestinal symptoms dominate the terminal course of untreated renal failure. Hiccoughing is an occasional and mysterious complication of uraemia which, if persistent, can exhaust and demoralize the patient. Peptic ulceration, perhaps due to the hypergastrinaemia of renal failure, occurs in about 20 per cent of patients. On barium meal most patients show giant rugal folds, the significance of which is unknown.

The Nervous System

Disorders of both central and peripheral nervous systems occur in uraemia. Peripheral neuropathy is rare and occurs in those whose renal failure has been present for a long time. The first symptom is of restless legs; the patients find that no position suits their legs for long and they always feel uncomfortable. This may sometimes coincide with the introduction of methyldopa and improves after the drug has been stopped. The next symptom to develop is a burning sensation in the feet. At this time no signs may be detectable, but nerve conduction studies show reduced velocity of conduction. Very rarely the neuropathy progresses to become totally incapacitating, involving both sensory and motor components.

The commonest symptoms of CNS involvement are drowsiness and lethargy. The patient is unable to concentrate and appears depressed. A coarse flap of the outstretched hands is common and muscular twitching can be seen even at rest. Terminally, the patient becomes more and more drowsy and indifferent until he lapses into coma. Grand mal seizures do occur, but they are usually associated with hypertension or intracerebral haemorrhage.

Muscular cramps are quite common and may be related either to sodium depletion (caused by either a salt-losing tendency or excessive use of diuretics), or to hypocalcaemia with acidosis.

Respiratory System

The lungs are spared any direct involvement, although at one time there was thought to be a specific 'uraemic lung'; this is probably the result of either pulmonary oedema or infection. Pulmonary thromboembolism may be less commonly associated with renal failure than other serious illnesses but does occur. Metabolic acidosis causes hyperventilation, which is particularly apparent in some patients with terminal uraemia or bicarbonate wasting. Bronchopneumonia is a common terminal event.

Blood

Anaemia is invariable in renal failure and its severity is approximately proportional to the degree of uraemia. Exceptions do occur, particularly in patients with polycystic kidneys who have a comparatively well maintained haemoglobin, while patients with analgesic nephropathy or mesangiocapillary glomerulonephritis are disproportionately anaemic. The red cells are normochromic and normocytic. The marrow appears paradoxically normal which is thought to be the main anomaly because anaemia should induce increased erythropoiesis.

This failure of stimulation is probably due to a lack of production of erythropoietin which is released from normal renal tissue in response to hypoxia, because serum levels of erythropoietin are reduced or undetectable in CRF. Erythropoietin acts on the marrow to increase production of red cells but has no effect on white cells or platelet production. Uraemic plasma has been found to have an inhibiting effect on the increase in erythropoiesis when erythropoietin is injected into polycythaemic animals. It is possible that an erythropoietin inhibiting factor is either produced or metabolized more slowly by diseased kidneys.

Other causes of anaemia are less important but some are more amenable to treatment. Blood loss from the bowel, haemolytic anaemia as the result of drugs (particularly methyldopa) or immunological mechanisms (as in SLE and mesangio-capillary nephritis) should be excluded. Uraemic red cells also have a reduced half-life in the circulation, and in some patients this is accentuated by increased splenic uptake which may be detected by appropriate isotopic studies.

Platelets are usually present in normal numbers in uraemia unless involved in the disease process, as they are in SLE, accelerated hypertension or the haemolytic uraemic syndrome. However, the function of platelets is affected by uraemia; both platelet aggregation and platelet Factor III release are abnormal, and these defects may contribute to the bruising apparent in advanced uraemia.

Neutrophil polymorphs are present in increased numbers in patients with uraemia but their function is also impaired. In vitro tests have shown defective chemotaxis and a less striking diminution in phagocytosis.

Lymphocyte counts are reduced in CRF and cell mediated immunity is seriously disordered as judged by both in vitro and in vivo tests; antibody production is less severely affected and secondary responses are probably normal. These defects suggest that patients with CRF would be particularly susceptible to infection, and, although there are no good studies to support this, it is widely believed to be true. In particular, it seems that tuberculosis and herpes infections are commoner among these patients.

The Skeletal System

Renal osteodystrophy is a common complication in renal failure in some areas, but in others it is hardly ever seen. The reason for this is unknown, but may reflect dietary habits, the chronicity of the disease and the age at which it develops. There are four main syndromes: secondary hyperparathyroidism, osteomalacia, soft tissue calcification and osteoporosis.

Secondary Hyperparathyroidism

Secondary hyperparathyroidism is the most common abnormality

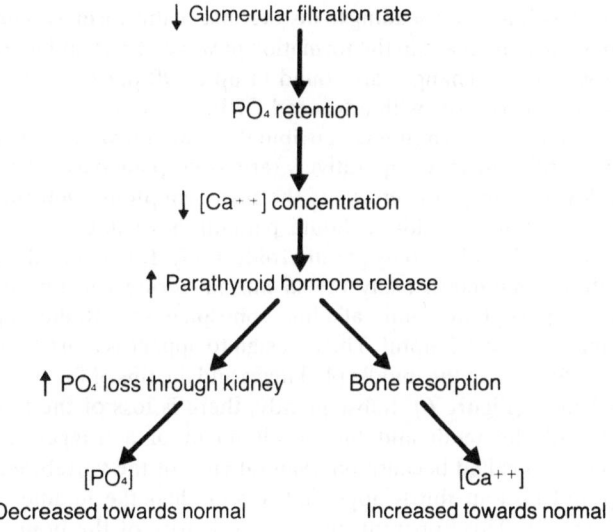

Figure 5. *Mechanism of development of secondary hyperparathyroidism in chronic renal failure. Eventually the effect of parathormone is insufficient to reduce the phosphate to normal. Serum calcium usually remains normal and PTH rises progressively.*

seen in most areas of Britain. It is caused by a high level of circulating parathyroid hormone produced by grossly hyperplastic glands, each of which may be 10 times the normal size. Experiments by Slatopolsky and his co-workers (1972) showed that dogs made chronically uraemic could be protected from the development of secondary hyperparathyroidism (as measured by a rise in parathyroid hormone concentration) by being fed a low phosphorus diet. The probable sequence of events is outlined in Figure 5.

Since raised parathyroid hormone concentrations are found in patients whose creatinine clearance is as high as 40 to 60 ml/min, the patient may have hyperparathyroidism for several years before renal failure becomes clinically evident. The effect of this hormone on bones is to cause reabsorption by an increase in osteoclastic activity, leading to disturbance of the normal architecture with an increase in the formation of woven bone and marrow fibrosis. These changes are found in up to 90 per cent of bone biopsies of patients with advanced CRF.

Fortunately, symptoms attributable to secondary hyperparathyroidism are comparatively rare. Bone pain, particularly of the lower limbs on exercise, is the main symptom. Deformities may develop in children. Some patients have intense pruritis which may be relieved by parathyroidectomy. Biochemical investigations characteristically reveal normal serum calcium and a raised phosphate and alkaline phosphatase. Radiographic changes are very helpful. The first sign to appear is a fuzziness of the radial side of the middle phalanges and the tips of the terminal phalanges (Figure 6). Subsequently, there is loss of the lamina densa of the teeth and the development of a 'rugger jersey spine'—so-called because on a lateral view of the vertebrae, the top and bottom thirds appeared denser than the middle third (Figure 7). This apparent increase in density of the bone may occur elsewhere and is called osteosclerosis. It is most common in children with renal failure.

Osteomalacia

Osteomalacia is difficult to detect until it is well advanced except

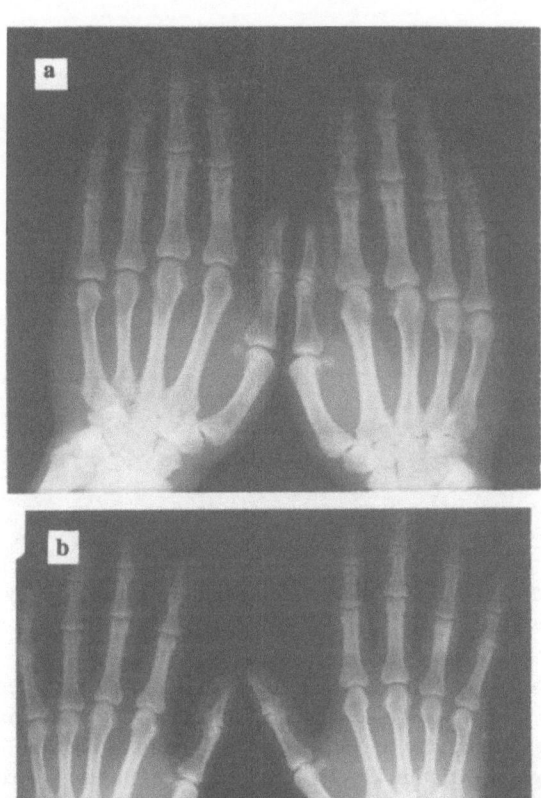

Figure 6. *Hand radiographs of a patient with chronic renal failure due to Alports syndrome. (a) In 1970, changes of hyperparathyroidism are visible. The radial edges of most of the middle phalanges are slightly irregular. (b) By 1977, the changes are gross and there is erosion of the tufts of the distal phalanges.*

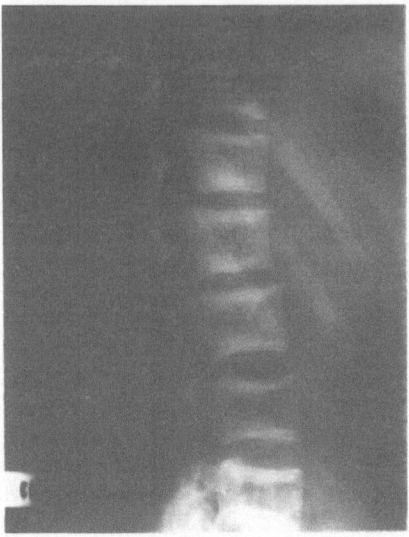

Figure 7. *Rugger jersey spine. The overall loss of bone density is also obvious.*

on bone biopsy. It is the result of failure to mineralize osteoid, so that on biopsy wide osteoid seams are seen. The abnormality is present in about 30 to 50 per cent of patients with CRF.

The parent vitamin D is cholecalciferol, but this is hydroxylated first in the liver to 25-hydroxycholecalciferol (25 OHD_3), and then in the kidney to 1,25-dihydroxycholecalciferol (1,25 $(OH)_2D_3$). This is by far the most potent form of vitamin D, and its actions are to increase calcium absorption from the gut and to promote bone mineralization secondary to the increased calcium levels. However, the direct effect of 1,25 $(OH)_2D_3$ on bone is to mobilize calcium and phosphate. By increasing the serum calcium level in the blood, 1,25 $(OH)_2D_3$ inhibits the production of para-thyroid hormone. In addition, it may have a direct suppressor effect on parathyroid hormone production, independent of serum calcium concentration. Failure of production of 1,25 $(OH)_2D_3$ by

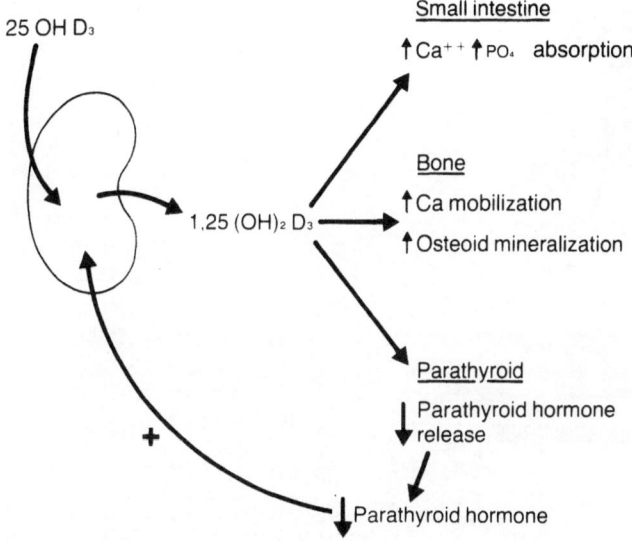

Figure 8. *Actions of vitamin D. Note that a reduction in circulating parathyroid hormone encourages the formulation of more 1,25(OH)$_2$D$_3$.*

the diseased kidney is thought to be the main cause of osteomalacia in renal failure and also contributes to the increased production of parathyroid hormone (Figure 8).

Clinically, although osteomalacia is a less common finding on bone biopsy, it is more likely to cause symptoms. The patient develops generalized aches, more marked in the legs and pelvis, which make walking painful. A proximal myopathy may be present causing difficulty with climbing stairs or getting out of chairs and even with combing hair. Bone tenderness is common. Children develop classical stigmata of rickets, genu valgum being the first abnormality, often before any pain occurs (Plate 6).

The serum calcium level is usually low, with a high phosphate and normal or elevated alkaline phosphatase. Radiographic changes develop late (Figure 9). Loss of bone density is the

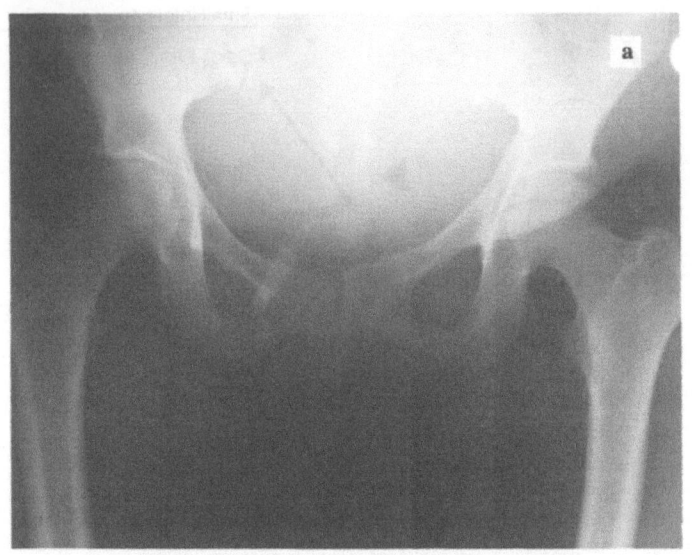

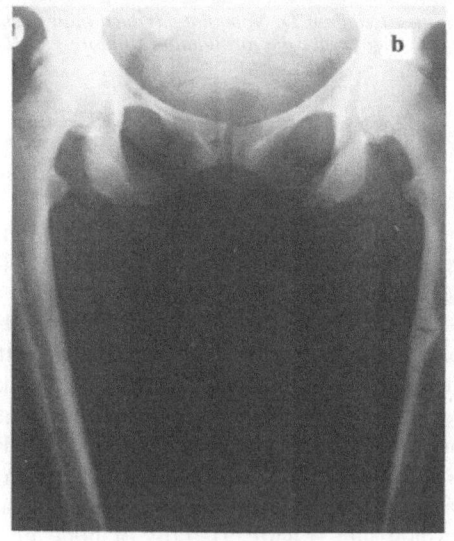

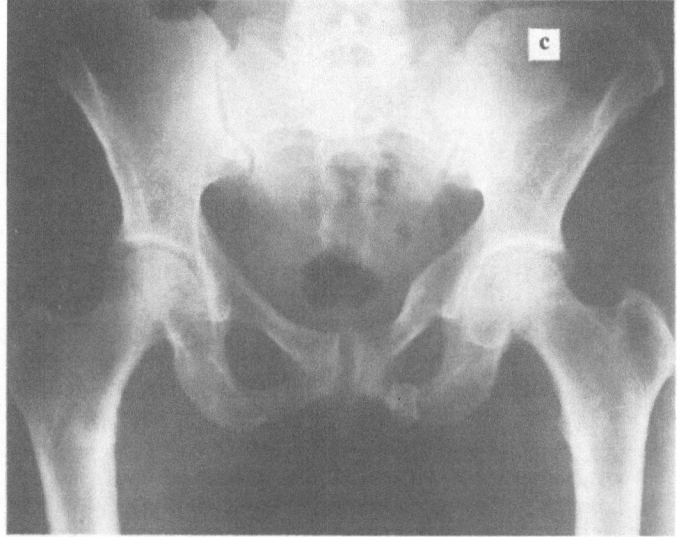

Figure 9. *(a) Pseudofracture. An early area of rarefaction is seen on the medial side of the shaft of the left femur. (b) Much grosser abnormality in the same area of the right femur. (c) Actual fracture of the right pubic ramus.*

earliest sign, but is difficult to interpret. The appearance of Looser's zones is always associated with severe pain and may be followed by pathological fractures.

Soft Tissue Calcification

Soft tissue calcification occurs when the serum calcium × phosphate product (in mmol/l) is persistently greater than 5.5 (or 70 when calcium and phosphate are measured in mg/dl). Calcification is first seen in arteries, particularly the ileal, but may extend to involve even small digital arteries (Figure 10a). Other soft tissues may become calcified; these include periarticular ligaments, the skin, cornea and conjunctiva (Figure 10b). Deposits in the skin may contribute to itching but clinically the most important deposits are those in the arteries because they con-

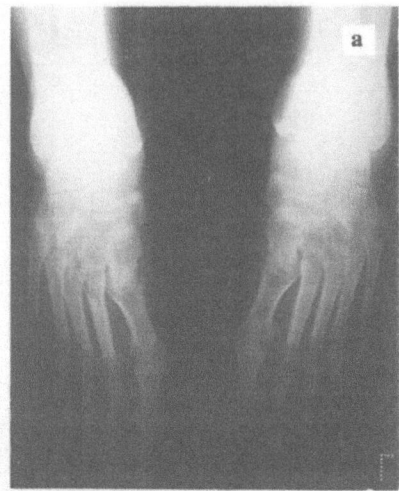

Figure 10. *Soft tissue calcification. (a) Note the circle of calcification between the first and second metatarsals of the left foot. This represents calcification in the dorsalis pedis artery and is one of the earliest sites of calcification. In the right foot more extensive arterial calcification is seen. (b) Note the calcification of soft tissues around the right shoulder.*

siderably increase the difficulty of forming arteriovenous fistulae which are necessary for regular dialysis treatment. Their role in the accelerated formation of atheroma is probably minor.

Osteoporosis

Osteoporosis refers to loss of bone mass and is found in some patients with renal failure. It is difficult to diagnose except through quantitative bone histology and its cause and clinical significance are unknown.

Although four varieties of renal osteodystrophy have been described, more than one type may be found in any one patient. Indeed, as already stated, osteomalacia is due to a lack of 1,25 $(OH)_2D_3$ which may also contribute to the rise in parathyroid hormone concentration (see Figure 8), thus increasing the calcium × phosphate product which leads to soft tissue calcification. By carefully monitoring the serum calcium, phosphate and alkaline phosphatase levels, and by taking radiographs of the hands at six-monthly intervals, it is possible to detect early changes. Bone biopsy is not routinely performed in all units, but it is particularly useful in the early diagnosis of osteomalacia. Management of these syndromes is discussed in Chapter 11.

References

Slatopolsky, E., Elkan, I. O., Weerts, C. & Bricker, N. S., Studies on the characterisation of the control system governing sodium excretion in uraemic man. *J. C. I.*, 1968, **47**, 521–530.

10. Investigation

Most patients who present with renal failure have no symptoms or signs referrable to the underlying process causing nephron destruction, but there are exceptions: patients with severe old pulmonary tuberculosis or chronic osteomyelitis may have amyloid; diabetics of 20 years' duration frequently develop diabetic nephropathy; a history of analgesic abuse is often significant; and bilateral loin masses strongly suggest polycystic renal disease. There are other examples in which the cause of renal failure may be apparent from a carefully taken history or physical examination, but the physician usually has to rely on other investigations to reveal the likely cause of renal failure, and in many patients the final diagnosis cannot be made with any certainty.

Proteinuria

The presence of more than 2 g of proteinuria in a 24 hour urine collection is often taken as an indication that chronic glomerulonephritis is the underlying disease. Chronic pyelonephritis is not usually associated with this degree of proteinuria, but a few patients with small scarred kidneys do have significant proteinuria. Such kidneys have been biopsied and they show some glomerular abnormalities, the significance of which remains unknown. A degree of proteinuria can occur in almost any cause of CRF, and it is therefore of little help in the differential diagnosis. However, massive proteinuria of more than 10 g/day is rare in patients with advanced renal failure and is often associated with focal glomerulosclerosis.

Intravenous Urography

The technique used to perform an adequate examination is the same as that described for ARF (see page 15). It is almost always possible to obtain satisfactory outlines of both kidneys, whatever the degree of renal failure. A reduction in size is the best indication that the patient's disease is chronic; even amyloid is frequently associated with small kidneys when renal failure is severe. Similarly, the presence of pericalyceal fat, seen as an unusual translucency around the calyceal cups, is typical of chronic disease. A difference in size between the kidneys suggests local causes, such as renal ischaemia, calculus nephropathy, chronic pyelonephritis or a congenital abnormality. Large kidneys with smooth irregularities of the calyces are characteristic of polycystic disease.

Chronic obstructive uropathy may be associated with kidneys of any size but the renal cortex is thinned and stretched around dilated calyces. A similar picture may sometimes be seen in patients with gross persistent vesicoureteric reflux; therefore, when found it is an indication for retrograde pyelography or a micturating cystogram.

Some patients with terminal renal failure have kidneys of normal or near normal size with smooth outlines. This appearance suggests a relatively short history and is most frequently seen in patients with glomerulonephritis or hypertension. The various changes found on intravenous urography in patients with renal failure are summarized in Table 15 and examples are shown in Figure 11.

Renal Biopsy

Renal biopsy is rarely of value in patients with chronic renal disease, as it is contraindicated if the kidneys are small or scarred.

Table 15. IVU changes in CRF.

Small kidneys with smooth outlines and normal calyces
Diffuse parenchymal disease—glomerulonephritis
                                    —diabetes
                                    —amyloid
Ischaemia affecting main renal artery
Senile atrophy
Hypoplasia
Longstanding hypertension

Small kidneys with smooth outlines and abnormal calyces
Longstanding obstruction
Papillary necrosis (rarely)
Longstanding vesico-ureteric reflux

Small kidneys with scarred outlines
Chronic pyelonephritis—deformed calyces
Papillary necrosis   —deformed calyces
Renal infarct   —normal calyces
Chronic tuberculosis
Radiation nephritis

N.B. These are the changes likely to be found in patients with advanced disease, and do not necessarily reflect appearances earlier in the natural history.

In these cases it is more difficult to obtain an adequate piece of tissue and to interpret the histological changes.

A final diagnosis may never be made with confidence in the majority of patients presenting with terminal renal failure, but it is important that reversible causes listed in Table 14 are excluded. An attempt should be made to ensure that the primary disease is unlikely to recur in a transplanted kidney. Several forms of glomerulonephritis have been reported to do so, including dense deposit disease (a form of mesangiocapillary glomerulonephritis), mesangial IgA disease and Goodpasture's syndrome, but the only disease which invariably and quickly causes renal failure in a transplanted kidney is oxalosis.

Other Investigations

In patients in whom it is not possible to make a firm diagnosis, the next objective is to look for factors which exacerbate or accelerate

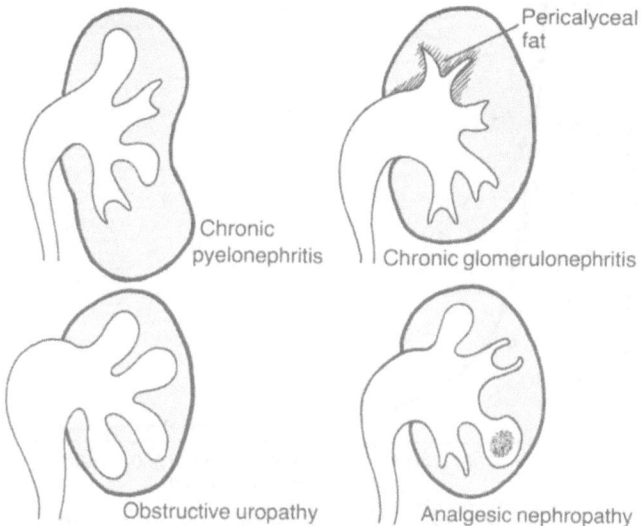

Figure 11. *IVU appearances in advanced renal failure.*

renal failure. These are relevant in any patient whatever the primary pathology, and when corrected should lead to improvement in renal function and symptoms. Obviously this has no effect on the underlying disease process but may improve the patient's wellbeing and is therefore worthwhile. The assessment of the progress of the disease requires both clinical and biochemical examination.

Tests of Renal Function

Creatinine clearance is the most accurate assessment of glomerular filtration which is routinely available. It does, however, have several inherent disadvantages. It is derived from the formula

$$\text{Creatinine clearance (ml/min)} = \frac{\text{UcV}}{\text{Pc}}$$

where Uc is the urinary concentration, and Pc the plasma concentration of creatinine. V is the volume of urine passed in a carefully

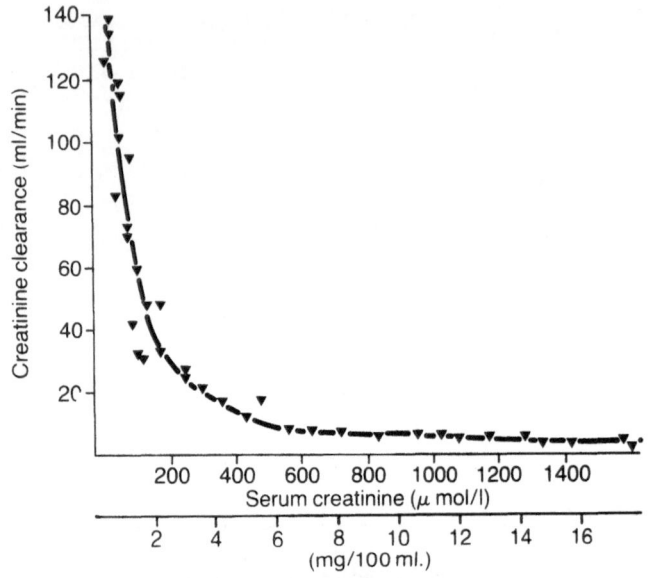

Figure 12. *Creatinine clearance versus serum creatinine.*

timed period (usually 24 hours) divided by the number of minutes in that period. The commonest inaccuracy is an incomplete urine collection. Creatinine clearance also overestimates the GFR because creatinine is secreted by the tubules and, since the amount secreted varies from person to person, it is impossible to arrive at an accurate value for GFR. Another cause of inaccuracy is that some methods of measuring serum creatinine are not entirely specific and therefore give a falsely high value.

Whatever its defects, the creatinine clearance remains the best routine clinical method of assessment of filtration function of the kidney until the disease is well advanced. Once the serum creatinine has risen above 300μmol/l (3.4 mg/dl), it alone is a sufficient guide. The reason is apparent from Figure 12, which shows that the serum creatinine rises very little until creatinine clearance has fallen to about 25 ml/min, thereafter it rises steeply and is of itself a sufficiently accurate reflection of changes in renal function.

Serum urea concentration is also routinely measured, but it reflects not only glomerular filtration but also protein intake and catabolism. The combination of urea and creatinine measurements is useful because the comparison between the two allows the detection of increased catabolism and an assessment of how well the patient is adhering to his diet (see below).

Estimations of the sodium, potassium, chloride and bicarbonate concentrations should be made regularly. It is important to realise that these are serum concentrations only, therefore hyponatraemia does not necessarily mean that the patient is salt depleted. In fact, mild hyponatraemia is most commonly seen in oedematous patients who have received large amounts of frusemide, but who still have an increase in their total body sodium. Pseudohyponatraemia is found in some patients with the nephrotic syndrome who have high serum lipid concentrations.

Both hypokalaemia and hyperkalaemia are of clinical importance but are rare. The former is usually seen in patients with secondary hyperaldosteronism or who are receiving large doses of diuretics or in those with a rare potassium-losing nephropathy. Hypokalaemia may aggravate renal failure and therefore should be corrected (see below). Severe hyperkalaemia is rare until renal failure is well advanced but mild hyperkalaemia is common, particularly in patients receiving a protein-restricted diet.

Acidosis is reflected in a reduced serum bicarbonate concentration. Renal failure is the most common cause of a large anion gap which is derived by adding chloride and bicarbonate concentrations and subtracting the total from the sodium concentration. The anion gap is normally less than 15 mmol/l but is considerably increased in renal failure, due to the retention of phosphate, sulphate and other anions which are not commonly measured. Therefore the anion gap reflects the degree of renal failure. If it is less than expected, then renal tubular acidosis should be suspected.

Other investigations which are routinely performed are the haemoglobin, calcium, phosphate, alkaline phosphatase and urate concentrations and urine culture. The patient's weight and blood pressure should also be recorded at each outpatient visit. Chest and hand radiography and an ECG are performed six monthly. It is also useful to ensure that the patient's hepatitis B surface antigen (Australia antigen) is negative at six-monthly intervals.

These investigations should give the clinician information on the individual patient's rate of progression towards renal failure, and any acceleration in that rate requires further investigation to determine its cause. There are several known factors which can cause such an acceleration.

11. Treatment

At this point it may be useful to re-emphasize the aims of treatment. These are:

1. To reverse the process causing renal parenchymal injury, which is rarely possible.

2. To slow the rate of progression to renal failure by correcting reversible factors.

3. To relieve the symptoms caused by advanced uraemia itself.

4. To assess the practicality of regular dialysis treatment and/or transplantation of an individual patient and to make this decision as early as possible so that it can be instituted while the patient remains fit. Dialysis and transplantation are discussed in Chapter 12.

Correction of Reversible Factors
Hypertension

Hypertension occurs in 80 per cent of patients with CRF, and adequate control of the blood pressure is perhaps the most important therapeutic measure to retard the rate of progression of uraemia. This is because there is a vicious cycle whereby parenchymal damage causes hypertension which in turn causes more structural changes, thus aggravating the hypertension. Although lowering the blood pressure leads to decreased flow through abnormal arterioles and therefore to reduction in glomerular filtration, this is transient and some recovery occurs as the arterial lesions resolve (see Figure 13). Therefore, hypoten-

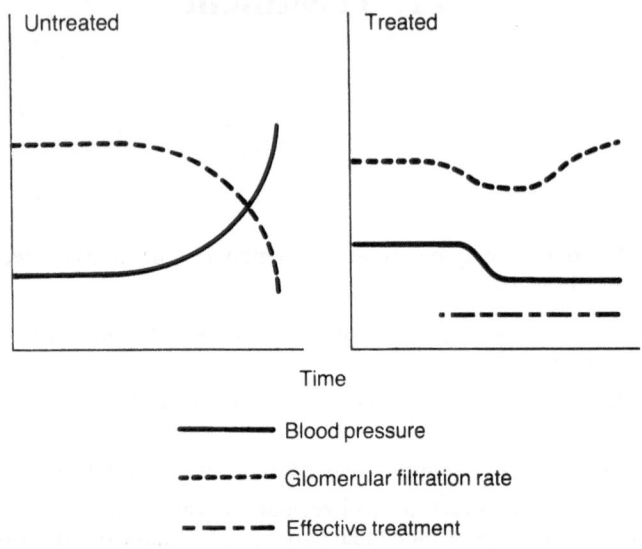

Figure 13. *Relationship between blood pressure, renal function and effect of treatment.*

sive therapy should be energetic. There are other benefits derived from adequate blood pressure control, e.g. the reduction in the incidence of strokes, left ventricular failure and the retardation in the development of atheroma.

Drug Therapy and Salt Restriction

There are two main therapeutic approaches: drug therapy and salt restriction. The former has become more effective with the introduction of new hypotensive agents, so that the need for an unappetising and severely salt-restricted diet is now rare. Each physician uses only a few of the many drugs now available. My own preference is for a combination of drugs in lower doses because, whereas the hypotensive effect is additive, the side effects are not.

A combination of β blocker and peripheral vasodilator is perhaps the most logical therapy, but unfortunately a really effective peripheral vasodilator free of severe side effects has yet to be found. Therefore, it is sensible to start with propranolol and increase the dose up to 240 mg/day before introducing a peripheral vasodilator. The maximal effect of propranolol may not be apparent for a few weeks until the reflex rise in peripheral vascular resistance has decreased. However, if the dose of 240 mg/day is ineffective, hydrallazine can be introduced and the dose increased up to 200 mg/day. The risk of a lupus-like reaction is increased if the dose is raised further. If the patient's blood pressure remains uncontrolled, methyldopa up to 2 g/day is sometimes effective. Most patients' hypertension is controlled by this regimen and propranolol can be increased further unless the standing pulse rate is less than 60/min.

However, if the patient has severe side effects or if the blood pressure control is inadequate, an alternative peripheral vasodilator can be used. Oral diazoxide is extremely effective, but may have to be used in doses which cause severe fluid retention (as do all peripheral vasodilators), hirsutism and hyperglycaemia, which may develop quite suddenly and be very severe. This last side effect is not common to minoxidol, which has yet to be released for general use in the UK. Minoxidol is very effective and appears to be well tolerated, particularly by male patients. The aim of therapy is to reduce the diastolic pressure below 95 mm Hg in patients up to 60 years of age. Even stricter control may be necessary in patients under 30 years or during pregnancy.

Other aspects of management are important. Women patients should be discouraged from taking a contraceptive pill and attention should be paid to fluid balance. Most drugs are more effective when total body sodium is normal or low. Therefore salt restriction is a useful adjunct to drug therapy, but it is rarely necessary to reduce the daily intake below 40 mmol (40 mEq), which most patients find acceptable if not palatable. Diuretics, particularly frusemide in doses up to 1 g/day, have proved effective in increasing urine volume and sodium loss. Side effects of large doses of frusemide are common and troublesome. In particular nausea and vomiting may force the patient to stop taking the drug and make it more difficult to take the other hypotensive agents. Recently a specific bullous eruption on the back of the hand has been reported in a few patients taking large doses of frusemide. However, it remains the most useful drug in controlling salt overload causing persistent hypertension.

Hypovolaemia

The problems of hypovolaemia are the reverse of those of hypertension and are most commonly found in patients whose disease primarily affects the renal tubules, e.g. chronic pyelonephritis, analgesic nephropathy, renal tubular acidosis or chronic obstructive renal disease, in which the capacity of the tubules to reabsorb sodium is reduced. This usually becomes apparent clinically when sodium is lost from the gastrointestinal tract or oral intake is abruptly reduced, as it is in patients who start vomiting or have severe nausea. The failing kidney is unable to adjust quickly to the changed circumstances, and sodium loss leads to hypovolaemia and a reduction in renal blood flow and, therefore, glomerular filtration.

The physical signs of hypovolaemia have been described (see page 7): loss of weight and postural hypotension are more easily elicited in patients with CRF and are relatively more important than other signs.

Hypovolaemia is corrected by intravenous replacement of saline or oral salt supplements, depending on the urgency. If the patient is not acidotic, sodium chloride given as Slow Sodium, 10 mmol (10 mEq) sodium/tablet, is a useful preparation. If acidosis is also present, sodium bicarbonate is more appropriate. Sodium replacement should continue until oedema or hypertension develops and then the dose reduced to a level which is consistent with normotension and the absence of oedema. This state constitutes the ideal fluid balance for that particular patient and is reflected by his weight, which should be noted and used as a reference point for future management. The improvement in renal function which may occur as a result of the correction of salt depletion may enable a patient with apparently terminal renal failure to live for one or two years more with few symptoms, depending on the underlying cause of renal failure.

Infection

Infection is the third of the important reversible factors in CRF, but it is not as significant as it is in ARF. The effect of infection on renal function may be very important and is always deleterious. The reasons for this are multifactorial and not fully understood. Fluid depletion due to increased insensible loss associated with fever, anorexia and vomiting are common. Infection also increases catabolism which raises the blood urea and aggravates uraemic symptoms, particularly vomiting and diarrhoea, which in turn leads to fluid depletion and more catabolism.

The types of infection and the organisms responsible are the same as in the general population, although urinary infections in patients with urinary tract abnormalities are particularly common. In some patients with gross abnormalities, such as an inoperable staghorn calculus, it may be impossible to sterilize the urine, and the main aim of therapy is to prevent recurrent bacteraemia.

In the treatment of other infections, the same restrictions on the use of antibiotics described in the management of ARF apply. In addition, nitrofurantoin and nalidixic acid are seldom used in advanced renal failure, the former because its main advantage is that it is concentrated in the urine, and this no longer occurs when the creatinine clearance falls below 50 ml/min and because it frequently provokes nausea and vomiting; and the latter because its toxic metabolites are normally excreted by the kidney. The second important aspect of treatment of infection is fluid replacement.

Drugs in Uraemia

When considering the administration of any drug to a uraemic patient, it is important to know what the kidney may do to the metabolism of the drug and what the drug may do to the metabolic state of the patient.

Renal Excretion of Drugs and Their Metabolism

Many drugs are excreted either wholly or partially by the kidney as the result of filtration or active tubular secretion. In patients with renal failure the risk of giving an inappropriately large dose is evident, and it is not surprising that 24 per cent of patients with a blood urea of more than 14 mmol/l (85 mg/dl) suffered an adverse drug reaction, compared to nine per cent of patients with normal renal function. This subject will not be reviewed in detail here but a few general principles and some examples are given:

1. Ensure that no unnecessary drugs are given. There should be a clear indication for the introduction of any drug and good evidence that it will improve the condition for which it is being given. This applies to any patient but the rule is frequently stretched. Such laxity is not appropriate in patients with renal failure and, in particular, sedatives, hypnotic and antidepressant therapy should be carefully planned.

2. If there is a choice between two drugs, one of which is not excreted by the kidney, then that drug should be chosen. If both drugs are excreted by the kidney, then the one with a greater difference between the therapeutic and toxic levels should be used. For example, penicillin derivatives are much safer than aminoglycosides in the treatment of infections.

3. The dose of the chosen drug may have to be modified. The initial or loading dose, i.e. that amount of drug required to produce an effective concentration throughout its volume of distribution, remains unaltered by renal failure. Thereafter, any drug excreted by the kidney should be given to patients with uraemia either less frequently or in a smaller amount than to patients with normal renal function. Many studies have been performed with numerous drugs which give some guidance and these should be consulted (see Table 5). However, serum levels should be checked if an assay is available, as clinical evidence of overdose may occur only after irreversible damage has occurred, e.g. with digoxin or gentamicin. If this is impossible, the clinician is forced to rely on his own observations and careful clinical follow-up is essential.

4. Administration of the drug should be stopped as soon as is practical.

If these rules are observed, almost any drug can be used in patients with advanced uraemia. The nearest to an exception is the tetra-cycline group.

Drug Effect on Uraemic Metabolism and Renal Function

The tetracyclines aggravate the uraemic state by raising blood urea in both normal and uraemic patients. Whereas this has little effect in patients with normal renal function, it may be cata-strophic in those with uraemia. Tetracycline inhibits normal pro-tein anabolism by preventing the incorporation of nitrogen into protein synthesis. Therefore, dietary nitrogen absorbed as amino-acids is catabolized directly to urea, and the patient's over-all nitrogen balance swiftly becomes negative. In CRF, nausea, vomiting and hypovolaemia develop, thus causing a true reduc-tion of renal function and a rise in serum creatinine. For this reason, all tetracyclines except doxycycline, whose anti-anabolic effect is least, should be avoided.

Papillary necrosis may be caused by analgesic abuse (see page 56). In patients who present with this syndrome and who have an underlying condition requiring analgesia, drugs containing phenacetin, aspirin and paracetamol should be avoided.

The treatment of hypertension is surprisingly little altered by renal failure, since any prolongation of the half-life of the drug will be reflected in the ease of blood pressure control. Therefore, the appropriate drug dose is that which controls the blood pressure without causing unacceptable side effects, and this can be titrated as in any other patient. It has been suggested that propranolol may cause a reduction in renal function, but the evidence is slim and the drug is still widely used.

Potassium in Renal Failure

Total body potassium is usually slightly reduced in patients with advanced renal failure. The reduction is proportional to the degree of acidosis, because hydrogen ions move into cells and displace an equivalent number of potassium ions. Tubular function, even in advanced renal failure, is surprisingly successful in excreting the displaced potassium. Therefore hyperkalaemia is usually mild, although the adaptive mechanism is stretched so that any catabolic stress may cause a sharp rise in serum potassium. Spironolactone should be avoided because it abolishes this protective mechanism. Protein restricted diets have a tendency to aggravate the mild hyperkalaemia but rarely to dangerous levels, so hyperkalaemia remains a comparatively minor problem in the management of most patients with slowly deteriorating renal function, unless they develop 'acute on chronic' renal failure.

The causes of hypokalaemia in patients with renal failure are listed in Table 16. The evidence that hypokalaemia adversely affects renal function is derived from animal experiments because it is never encountered in patients who do not have hypertension, infection, hypovolaemia or obvious renal disease. However, its correction is considered one of the measures capable of improving renal function, but it is rare in clinical practice.

The reduced total body potassium found in advanced uraemia may be one of the causes of insulin resistance found in these patients, as both are reversed by periods of regular dialysis treatment.

Hypercalcaemia

Hypercalcaemia is a rare cause, rather than a consequence, of renal failure. It may also result from an overdose of vitamin D or its analogues. Of the symptoms which it produces, the most

Table 16. Causes of hypokalaemia associated with renal failure.

Loss from the gastrointestinal tract

Diuretic overdose

Secondary hyperaldosteronism, e.g. accelerated hypertension

Renal tubular acidosis

Correction of acidosis without K^+ replacement

important in the uraemic patient are nausea and vomiting leading to hypovolaemia and further deterioration of renal function. It also increases the calcium × phosphate product, thus increasing soft tissue deposition in various organs including the kidney, with consequent acceleration of renal failure. The correct treatment is to remove the cause and to correct hypovolaemia.

Hyperuricaemia

The serum uric acid concentration increases as renal function fails. Since it is known that primary hyperuricaemia due to an enzyme deficiency is a cause of renal failure, it has been postulated that secondary hyperuricaemia due to CRF may accelerate the decline of renal function. There is one important difference, in that primary hyperuricaemia is associated with hyperuricosuria, and it is this which leads to the tubular and interstitial crystal formation which is the stimulus for the inflammatory reaction that causes renal parenchymal damage. The hyperuricaemia of CRF occurs because of decreased urinary urate excretion and, therefore, crystals are not deposited in the kidney. Thus it is theoretically unlikely that reducing the serum urate will decrease the rate of development of renal failure. One study, which used allopurinol to reduce the serum urate, supports this conclusion. Therefore, unless values in excess of 750 mmol/l (12 mg/dl) are found, there seems little point in attempting to lower the serum urate. Values above this level are seldom found in CRF.

Clinical attacks of gouty arthritis are rare in patients with CRF although they have been described, especially in patients with lead nephropathy or polycystic kidneys. The reason for this is unknown and somewhat surprising in view of the high urate concentration. One possible explanation is that abnormal polymorph neutrophil function prevents the normal phagocytosis of urate crystals and therefore release of polymorph lysosomal enzymes which cause the acute inflammation of gout.

Obstruction

Obstruction may itself lead to CRF or may complicate the course of renal failure from other causes, such as polycystic kidneys, analgesic nephropathy, tuberculosis, or polyarteritis nodosa. It is important to ensure that any patient with CRF does not have an obstructive element to that failure.

The diagnosis is usually made on the IVU appearances. The more chronic the obstruction, the more probable that the ureter will be dilated and convoluted.

Relief of obstruction usually requires surgical correction. However, in patients who have undergone several operations for stones, strictures or retroperitoneal fibrosis, it may be difficult to assess whether the IVU changes are functionally significant or merely the result of an obstruction that has been adequately relieved. Other patients may have large renal pelves of no urodynamic significance. If renal failure is not advanced, these may be detected by the administration of frusemide during the IVU, and if the pelvis does not dilate by more than 25 per cent in the subsequent diuresis, then the appearances are unlikely to be significant and the patient may be saved an unnecessary operation.

The decision on whether to operate is usually straightforward but in some patients may be extraordinarily difficult: the guiding rule is that the operation should be designed to save nephron function rather than to alter the appearances of an IVU. In particular, an operation should not be undertaken for loin pain unless it is certain that the dilatation seen on the IVU is of urodynamic significance, because it is unlikely that it will relieve the patient's symptoms or protect renal function.

Treatment of Uraemia and its Complications

Diet

The introduction of a protein restricted diet by Giordano in 1963 and Giovanetti in 1964 and its modification for British tastes by Berlyne and Shaw (1965) has completely changed the clinical syndrome of terminal renal failure.

The rationale for this diet is that it provides as much nitrogen as is needed to maintain nitrogen balance, and minimizes the intake of 'unusable' dietary nitrogen. It also aims to encourage the re-use of endogenous urea. These three factors are inter-related, so that to determine the overall value of one, the other two factors have to be kept constant, and an adequate calorie intake from other sources has to be assured.

In order to minimize unusable dietary nitrogen, the quality of protein in the diet must be improved. High quality protein is that which leads to the lowest urinary urea excretion because the greatest proportion of the constituent amino acids have been used in the production of endogenous protein. Egg and milk protein have the highest biological value for man.

The degree to which endogenous urea (broken down by bacteria in the colon to ammonia, which is then absorbed and available for protein synthesis) is used remains a matter for conjecture. It is possible that it provides about 2 g of nitrogen/day and could, therefore, further reduce dietary protein requirement. Sufficient dietary calories other than protein must be provided to maintain nitrogen balance, unless the patient is obese. In patients of normal weight, about 35 to 50 cal/kg/day should be provided, depending on the patient's activity. If 50 per cent of the requirement is given as carbohydrate, there may be some reduction in triglyceride and cholesterol concentrations which are commonly elevated in uraemic patients.

What Can Diet Achieve?

Protein restricted diets have been remarkably successful in controlling the gastrointestinal symptoms of uraemia. Nausea, anorexia, vomiting and diarrhoea are all quickly improved. The patient's foetor disappears and his sense of wellbeing improves. Haemoglobin may rise because of increased survival of red cells in the peripheral circulation. (There is no evidence of increased marrow activity.) Pruritus may also be relieved, although in the occasional patient very severe protein restriction may be required to achieve this.

The diet has little or no effect on renal osteodystrophy, peripheral neuropathy, pericarditis or hypertension. There is a tendency for the serum potassium to rise, even though the total body potassium remains low.

Therefore, correct dietary management prolongs the symptom-free period of declining renal function and may also prolong life, since intractable vomiting and diarrhoea lead to hypovolaemia and accelerated reduction in renal function.

Practical Steps

The degree of renal function at which individual patients experience symptoms varies a great deal. Since protein restriction is unwelcome to most patients and since its effect is to relieve symptoms rather than to improve renal function, it should not be introduced until the patient can be expected to derive benefit. Specifically, it should not be used simply to improve biochemical results, although most patients experience symptoms when their blood urea is about 35 mmol/l (200 mg/dl).

The diet chosen should be designed for an individual patient; the tastes of Indians are very different from those of Highlanders from Skye, and a dietician's advice should be sought to accommodate the individual's tastes. The following are intended as guidelines:

1. Protein content. It is important to ensure that the patient is not subject to prolonged net nitrogen loss. Various studies have shown that between 0.25 and 0.5 g protein/kg body weight/day are required to maintain nitrogen balance. The higher the biological value of the protein in the diet, the lower the total necessary protein intake. The protein of milk and eggs has a very high biological value, but a diet of milk, eggs, fats and carbohydrates is boring when taken over several months, and the recent trend has been to give 0.5 g of protein/kg body weight/day and to include meat, normal bread and vegetables in the diet. Thus a 70 kg patient should receive between 30 and 40 g of protein/day. If he has significant proteinuria, this should also be added to the dietary requirement.

If the patient's symptoms remain uncontrolled, dialysis should be started. However, if this form of treatment is not available, or if it is contraindicated, then further protein restriction to 20 g/day, using a high quality protein diet, may help. Special protein-free flour has been produced from which bread, cakes or biscuits can be baked to help make up the calorie requirement. Almost all meat, fish and vegetables are eliminated. This will only be tolerated if the patient receives obvious benefit and should, therefore, be commenced in hospital.

2. Calorie content. For reasons given above between 35 and 50 cal/kg/day should be provided.

3. Vitamin supplements. These have been routinely prescribed in many units, but there is little likelihood of any deficiency occurring, provided a properly balanced 40 g protein diet is given. It is wise to supply such supplements with more restricted protein diets. Methionine supplements which were originally given with the modified Giovanetti diet are no longer thought to be necessary.

4. Amino acid and α keto acid diets. It has been shown that amino acids alone, when given in the correct proportions, are an adequate source of nitrogen. Suitable preparations of the amino acids are available as tablets, e.g. Kidnamin, about 80 of which must be taken each day. Calories are provided by cream, Hycal and other pure fat or carbohydrate sources. The diet is not appetizing, but patients with no renal function have been managed on these diets with the aid of very infrequent peritoneal dialyses. Some patients with intractable pruritus actually welcome this type of diet because it causes relief of their symptoms. α keto acids have also been used because they are transaminated with ammonia, which is provided by the breakdown of urea in the colon, to produce amino acids, thus causing an even greater reduction in urea. However, these diets are seldom used outside research institutions.

5. The salt and fluid requirements. These depend on the patient's urinary sodium loss and blood pressure. The principles of management have already been outlined.

Once a patient has been started on a protein restricted diet, it is possible to check the success with which he is managing it by comparing the creatinine/urea ratio. This should be greater than 35 when the creatinine is measured in μmol/l and the urea in mmol/l. The equivalent formula for values expressed in mg/dl is a urea/creatinine ratio of less then 20. If the patient continues to have symptoms such as nausea, vomiting or anorexia, and if this ratio is found to be unsatisfactory, then the patient is either catabolic or has not adhered to his diet.

Renal Osteodystrophy

The symptoms of renal bone disease can almost always be alleviated effectively by the following measures:

1. Oral phosphate binders. Aluminium hydroxide can be taken as either a liquid, capsule or tablet with food. It is important that it is actually mixed with the food in order to bind dietary phosphate, thus preventing its absorption. Since phosphate is mainly contained in protein, the amount ingested is reduced when the protein intake is restricted. The aim of this therapy is to maintain the serum phosphate at about 2 mmol/l. If it is reduced too much over a prolonged period, hypophosphataemic rickets may ensue. However, the main disadvantage of this therapy is the extreme distaste with which most patients view it; 60 ml aluminium hydroxide gel or 12 Alucaps each day is a formidable amount and often induces nausea so that some compromise in the dose is often necessary.

By decreasing phosphate absorption, the serum phosphate is. partially controlled, which decreases both the production of parathyroid hormone and ectopic phosphate deposition thus, perhaps, retarding the progress of renal failure. If the patient has a raised alkaline phosphatase, aluminium hydroxide therapy should be used first in an attempt to reduce it towards normal, and this is often successful.

2. Vitamin D therapy. Recently 1 α hydroxycholecalciferol (1 α OHD$_3$) has been released for general use in the UK. This has established itself as the choice form of vitamin D to be used in renal failure, because it can be readily hydroxylated at the 25 position in the liver to form 1,25 (OH)$_2$D$_3$. It is remarkably active and the dose range lies between 1 μg $\times$ 2 per week and 3 μg/day. The dose for each patient has to be titrated against symptoms, biochemical changes and radiological abnormality. The therapy leads to mineralization of osteoid seams and to a reduction in parathyroid hormone production, to an extent that in some patients it causes a 'medical parathyroidectomy'. Thus 1 α OHD$_3$ can be expected to raise the serum calcium, lower the alkaline phosphatase and heal lesions radiologically.

The main limitation to its use, as with all forms of vitamin D, is hypercalcaemia, which may accelerate renal failure and make it impossible to give an adequate dose. Fortunately the hypercalcaemia caused by this form of vitamin D is reversed within one to two weeks of stopping therapy, compared with up to 12 weeks with the more conventional preparations. Most patients with renal osteodystrophy can be managed with a combination of phosphate binder and 1 α OHD$_3$. Their symptoms are quickly relieved and both biochemical and radiological abnormalities can be improved and usually alleviated completely.

3. Partial parathyroidectomy. This is rarely necessary in patients with CRF, although it is more frequently required once dialysis has been started. The main indication is severe hyperparathyroidism causing symptoms of bone pain and/or bony deformity which are not relieved by the methods already described. It should be performed by a surgeon who has experience of the procedure, because of the unpredictable anatomy of the four glands. Patients should start 1 α OHD$_3$ 1 μg/day one week before the operation at which all parathyroid glands should be identified, the task being made easier by the gross hypertrophy which is usual. Either 3 or 3$\frac{1}{2}$ of these hypertrophic glands should be removed.

Postoperative care is critically important; serum calcium, electrolytes, urea and creatinine should be measured regularly, at least three times in the first 24 hours. Catastrophic hypocalcaemia is rare if the patient is properly premedicated with $1 \alpha OHD_3$ and if only a partial parathyroidectomy is performed. Even so, intravenous calcium may have to be given. Care should be taken not to correct acidosis unless hypocalcaemia has been corrected, otherwise the patient may suffer convulsions. Basal atelectasis is particularly common and routine chest physiotherapy should be started within 24 hours of the operation. $1 \alpha OHD_3$ therapy should be continued unless hypercalcaemia develops. Relief of bone pain can be achieved quickly, and there should be a progressive improvement in the biochemical and radiographic abnormalities.

Anaemia

The anaemia of CRF is intractable to treatment but may be exacerbated by other factors which should always be searched for and corrected. Iron deficiency is sometimes present and is best detected by staining a marrow smear for iron or measuring the plasma ferritin, because the usual indices of iron deficiency (e.g. plasma iron concentration, iron binding capacity, mean corpuscular volume and mean corpuscular haemoglobin content) are not always reliable. Infections and some drugs may also aggravate the anaemia, as may some underlying immunological processes.

Specific measures to increase marrow activity, such as cobalt or anabolic steroid administration, have been tried with some success, but their toxic effects are such that their use is not widespread. Undoubtedly an effective treatment for the anaemia of CRF would radically improve the patient's wellbeing, but such a remedy has yet to be found.

12. Dialysis and Transplantation

The assessment of a patient for replacement therapy by regular dialysis or transplantation is an essential part of the management of advanced renal failure. The earlier a decision can be made, the more likely it is that a smooth transfer will be achieved. Unfortunately, the scarcity of resources and the unevenness of their distribution in countries and between regions of a single country mean that each nephrologist has his own criteria and methods for the assessment of individual patients which he considers most equitable for his own district's needs.

Before spelling out how admission policies are practised, it is worth giving a brief description of what is offered by the various forms of replacement therapy. Dialysis and transplantation will be dealt with separately, but it should be realized that most patients start with dialysis and are subsequently transplanted, and if that transplanted kidney fails, they are taken back onto a dialysis programme (see Figure 14).

Dialysis

Access

Regular dialysis treatment became possible with the discovery that arteriovenous silastic shunts could be maintained for some months. Since 1968, this external synthetic shunt has been superseded by the Cimino fistula, a subcutaneous end-to-side or side-to-side arteriovenous anastomosis usually between the radial artery and an adjacent vein (Plate 7). The injection of blood at

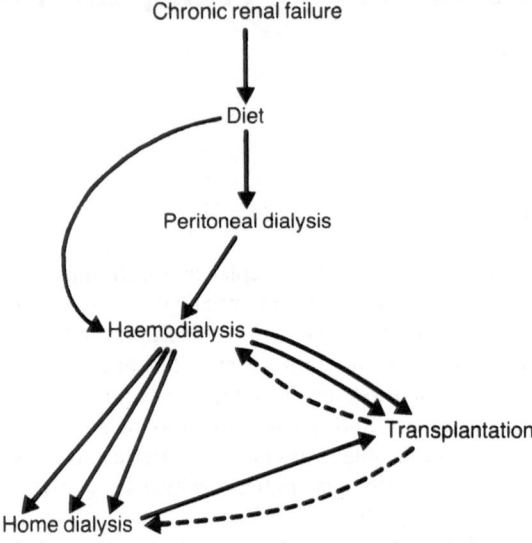

Figure 14. *Treatment of end stage renal failure. Note that home dialysis and transplantation are two forms of treatment which can cope with a continuing increase in the number of patients.*

arterial pressure directly into the forearm veins causes them to dilate and their walls to hypertrophy over the following weeks (Figure 15). These enlarged veins can be cannulated at each dialysis and blood pumped out in sufficient quantity (200 to 350 ml/min) to achieve a satisfactory dialysis. Between dialyses, the needles are withdrawn rendering the patient 'waterproof', so that he can swim or bathe at will, which those patients with the silastic shunts are not able to do. The risk of infection is also dramatically reduced, and the life of the fistula is two or three times that of the shunt. For these reasons less than 10 per cent of patients are now dialysed through shunts which are only used when all else fails.

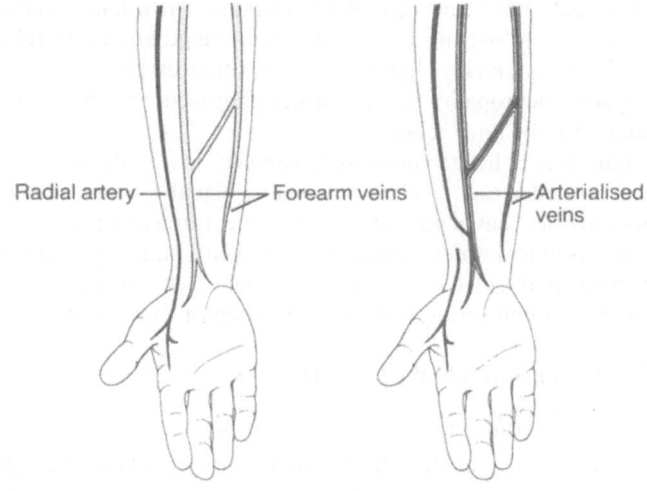

Figure 15. *Cimino fistula. Diagram shows an end-to-side anastomosis between the radial artery and a neighbouring vein. Over the next six weeks these veins hypertrophy, dilate and become more tortuous. They can then be used as shown in Plate 7.*

What Does Dialysis Do?

It is not the intention of this book to describe the physical or technical principles of dialysis, but to review its clinical achievements and failures. The main role of dialysis is to replace the excretory function of the kidney by diffusion of molecules across a semipermeable membrane, such as cellophane or cuprophane. It removes many of the nitrogenous waste products of metabolism, some drugs and excess potassium, corrects acidosis, and extracts water by ultrafiltration. None of these functions are performed with the same efficiency as is achieved by normal renal function. Also dialysis is intermittent rather than continuous.

The correction achieved in the biochemical environment allows the patient to lose most of his uraemic symptoms. Pericarditis usually heals quickly, hypertension is often easier to control, peripheral neuropathy may be slowly improved, and the itching patient usually finds relief.

Dialysis does little to improve anaemia or to heal the lesions of renal osteodystrophy. Hypertension is actually aggravated in about five per cent of patients, and becomes refractory to removal of fluid (salt and water) or hypotensive agents until nephrectomy has been performed. These patients almost always have enormously elevated serum renin and angiotensin concentrations.

What Does it Mean to the Patient?

Time Spent on Machine

There has been a steady reduction in the number of hours thought necessary for patients to spend on the machine each week. In 1970 it was common for them to endure 28 hours, whereas now 12 to 15 hrs/week is the rule, even though there has been no radical change in the technology of dialysis during that time (Plate 8). Obviously patients welcome any reduction and further trials are under way, but even at 12 hours/week, fluid and, therefore, blood pressure control is less easy, and patients tend to be more anaemic. The maximum time that patients can go without dialysis varies according to their residual renal function, diet and serum potassium. As a general rule, few patients can survive more than five days off dialysis, and this has considerable implications both for them and their families. Thus no holidays abroad or prolonged visits to their friends are possible, and this constitutes a considerable loss of freedom. Exchange visits between dialysis units, portable dialysis machines (such as the Redy machine) and holiday caravan dialysis stations may lighten this load somewhat.

Diet and Fluid Restriction

Diet on dialysis is better than for patients with CRF because protein restriction is virtually eliminated. A daily allowance of 60 g of protein allows most patients to enjoy considerable freedom. However, this gain in freedom is more than offset by the care that most patients have to observe with their fluid and potassium restrictions. The basic fluid allowance is 500 ml/day due to insensible loss, but this can be augmented if the patient is lucky enough to continue to pass urine. Even so a fluid allowance of more than 1 litre/day is unusual. The consequences of overindulgence may be uncontrolled hypertension, peripheral oedema and sometimes frank pulmonary oedema. Therefore, most patients come to understand the rationale from bitter experience. The social implications of restricting fluid intake to 500 ml or 1 pt a day are considerable, and most patients stretch it as far as they dare.

Potassium restriction is essential and without renal function, natural wastage is minimal. The consequences of hyperkalaemia are ventricular fibrillation and sudden death. High potassium foods, such as chips, chocolates, fruits and nuts, are among the simple and otherwise harmless delicacies of life and their removal from the diet particularly upsets some patients.

Water soluble vitamins are removed by dialysis and blood losses, although small, may cause iron deficiency. Therefore, oral folic acid, vitamins B and C and iron supplements are routinely given. Aluminium hydroxide preparations are also required for reasons already detailed.

Dialysis and Employment

It cannot be stressed often enough that dialysis is a way of life and not a state of suspended life in which the patients wait for something, perhaps a transplant, to come along. This must be repeated to patients, their families and sometimes their employers and family doctors as well. Certainly the obstacles dialysis patients have to overcome in order to stay at work are greater than those of the normal person, especially at a time or in an area of high unemployment.

It is easier if the patient is dialysed in the evening, either at home or in the hospital, but home dialysis offers greater flexibility. Thus the European data of 1978 shows that 36 per cent of patients on hospital dialysis were employed full-time compared with 64 per cent of patients on home dialysis. Therefore, home dialysis appears to offer much better opportunities for employment, although it is probable that many centres select the more employable patients for home dialysis. It is also true that many patients suffer financially, even if they stay at work, through failure to work overtime, failure to be promoted, inability to travel and lack of flexibility, all of which are the direct consequences of dialysis.

Dialysis and the Family

Most patients live with their families and rely on them for support and affection which is crucial to their wellbeing. The demands made on members of the family, particularly the spouse (or parents of children on dialysis) are considerable, even when dialysis is actually performed in the hospital. A husband or wife who also has to help in setting up the machine, dialysing the patient, stripping the machine, coping with emergencies and performing some of the functions that would have been expected of the patient had they been in better health, is more exposed to anxiety and stress and enjoys less freedom than in normal households. Wives of patients can spend less time on housework or in looking after the children, and husbands of patients may have to take over many of the maternal roles within the family and have less time to devote to work. Studies have shown that marriages which were stable before dialysis cope surprisingly well, whereas those that were unsound tend to become even more so. This is obviously important to the preliminary assessment.

The Psychology of Dialysis

The preceding paragraphs have perhaps concentrated on the disadvantages of dialysis. There are real problems which have to be and are regularly overcome by both patients and their families. The starting point, terminal renal failure, is one from which most people are grateful to escape alive. If dialysis is portrayed as a way of life with its own rules and the reasons behind those rules explained, then patients will frequently accept the situation.

If dialysis goes well, a patient may expect to feel about 80 per cent of normal wellbeing and many enjoy much better health than they did during the period of renal failure; indeed some insist that they have not felt better for years. Providing they can adapt their way of life, they will remain content. It is patients who are unable to accept the limitations imposed who are prone to bouts of despair. These are the patients for whom a successful transplant seems to offer the perfect solution, and this may well be so.

Of course, not all patients fall in these two groups, nor are the reasons for dissatisfaction always so readily identifiable. Some patients are worn down by a succession of minor accidents, such as a clotted fistula, poorly controlled hypertension or recurrent infections. Yet the majority of patients are able to lead a life which exploits the possibilities available; some make few concessions to their condition and never even tell their friends or workmates that they are regularly dialysed and these friends regard then as entirely normal.

The Cost of Dialysis

Computing the cost to the health authorities of one patient kept on dialysis is difficult. A recent study (Rennie, *New England Journal of Medicine*, 1978, **298**, 372) suggests that each patient on hospital dialysis costs about \$24,500 a year (£13,000) and \$15,400 (£8,000) on home dialysis. These figures are probably directly comparable to the cost in Britain, where a higher proportion of patients are on home dialysis (66 per cent) than in any other country.

The Success of Dialysis

Patient survival on dialysis is now quite good; about 90 per cent are alive at one year, 80 per cent at two years and thereafter there is a mortality of about 5 to 10 per cent per year. Patients with systemic disease, such as diabetes, survive less well. One of the major causes of death is from vascular accidents, such as myocardial infarctions. The survival of patients on home dialysis is generally slightly better than on hospital dialysis (70 per cent versus 55 per cent at 5 years).

Patient Selection

It should be possible to deduce from the foregoing description which patients should be ideally suited to dialysis, but few patients are ideal and the manner in which selection is made varies from unit to unit. Since Britain has only one unit per million of the population, most patients must be placed on home dialysis. It is almost always possible to arrange for the conversion of a room in the house or the installation of a Portakabin in the garden or for the family to move to a more suitable house. Home dialysis is impractical if patients do not have the support of their families. Since survival is better in the younger age groups, most units have an upper age limit of 60 years but this also reflects the availability of resources. In Norway the average age on admission is 53 years; in the UK it is 39 years. The patient himself must be well motivated, which is the rule, and have a stable personality.

It is also a considerable advantage if the patient can speak the same language as that of the staff on whom he will depend. Given sufficient resources there are few patients who would not be able to get by on dialysis, and it is the nephrologist's unfortunate task to have to compare various patients' suitability. Provision of adequate resources rests with the decisions of administrators and politicians on whom many competing claims are made for the available money.

The Non-nephrologist and Dialysis Patient

It is difficult for general practitioners, or even hospital doctors other than nephrologists, to gain experience in the problems of management of patients on dialysis, since there are only about 70 to 140 per million of the population affected. Yet any doctor may be involved in an emergency involving such a patient. The following are some simple rules of management:

1. Most dialysis patients have a clear idea of the do's and don't's of their management. Furthermore they are not reluctant to express their opinion to the doctor looking after them. It is often wise to take their advice, unless there is a clear indication to the contrary.

2. Fluid overload is a common complication and may present as peripheral oedema, hypertension, or even pulmonary oedema. For this reason, if the dialysis patient suffers a common emergency

such as myocardial infarction or a gastrointestinal haemorrhage, it is unsafe to put up an intravenous line and keep it open with one or two litres of fluid/24 hours. Hypertension can be treated acutely by the intravenous infusion of hydrallazine or diazoxide in the normal way, but the presence of pulmonary oedema is an indication for immediate dialysis.

3. Hyperkalaemia is a great hazard and care should be taken to avoid giving potassium supplements in any form, some of which may not be obvious (for example, bran or a potassium salt of penicillin). If the patient is severely hypokalaemic due to persistent diarrhoea, then potassium supplements may be indicated but their use should be carefully controlled. The serum potassium should be checked as soon as the patient is admitted and hyperkalaemia is an indication for early dialysis.

4. Vascular access. Most patients have a Cimino fistula in the forearm. Its patency should be checked, particularly if the patient is hypotensive or hypovolaemic, and this is easily done by noting the presence of a thrill over the site of the anastomosis. Venepuncture should not be performed on this arm.

5. Infection. Patients on haemodialysis do have a slightly increased incidence of infection which may be more serious than in the normal population because of the impaired defence mechanisms. Infection of the fistula site is particularly dangerous because of potential septicaemia. Even a small local infection there should be treated seriously.

6. Drug therapy should be modified to reflect the complete absence of renal function.

7. It is a good rule to inform the unit to which the patient is attached of any development and to seek their advice on the best management as early as possible.

Transplantation

A successful transplant is the dream of almost all patients with terminal renal failure. The fact that not all share the dream is due to the risk involved.

Benefits of a Successful Transplant

When functioning satisfactorily, all the complications of uraemia are reversed; the patient's haemoglobin returns to normal, bones heal, neuropathy is corrected and they are free of the fluid and dietary restrictions. Even passing urine becomes an ecstatic experience to be savoured again and again. It is no wonder that most patients eagerly accept the gamble.

Risks Involved

The risks are equally dramatic. Although the transplant operation itself is comparatively safe, many patients, perhaps 12 per cent, die when the transplant fails, mainly through infection. Rejection of the graft occurs in many more patients, so that only 45 per cent of grafts received from unrelated cadaver donors are functioning at the end of two years and 35 per cent at five years. Unfortunately, it remains impossible to predict the outcome before transplantation. HLA typing has been disappointing to the extent that some units no longer attempt to match grafts preoperatively. The morbidity associated with transplantation is also high and is due to the long-term use of prednisolone and azathioprine to prevent rejection. The patients are usually mildly Cushingoid in appearance, subject to infections and have a higher incidence of gastrointestinal haemorrhage and avascular necrosis of various bones. There is also a slightly increased risk of malignancy, particularly involving the reticuloendothelial system.

It is these difficulties that have persuaded the nephrologists of some countries, particularly Italy and Germany, to make long-term dialysis the treatment of choice. However, transplantation can be dramatically successful and even if rejection occurs, the patient is usually able to restart regular dialysis.

The chances of success are much greater if the kidney from a closely related donor is used, 75 per cent functioning at two years and 70 per cent at five years. Naturally, performing an operation on a perfectly fit person is distasteful to some, but is justifiable if the donor is well motivated and every care is taken to ensure success. It is certainly less stressful to many families than to have to support a relative on regular dialysis over several years. Transplantation allows more patients with terminal renal failure to be treated, and this is extremely important in areas where insufficient dialysis resources are available.

Kidney Donor Cards

Every member of the public can contribute to this programme by carrying a kidney donor card and making their wishes known to their nearest relatives. Every member of the medical profession can help by considering a patient with brain damage as a possible donor of two kidneys. Undoubtedly the cheapest way of providing an adequate service to patients with terminal renal failure is a sufficient supply of cadaver donors, and this rests with the legislators, the public and members of the medical profession.

References

Rennie, D., Home dialysis and the costs of uraemia, *New Engl. J. Med.*, 1978, **298**, 399.

Further Reading

Rennie, D., Home dialysis and the costs of uraemia. *N. Engl. J. Med.*, 1978, **297**: 399–400.
Schoenfeld, P. I. and Humphreys, M. H., A general description of the uraemia state. In: *The Kidney.* Brenner, B. M. and Rector, F. C. (Eds.) London, Philadelphia: W. B. Saunders Co. Ltd., 1976, Ch. 33, 1423–47.
Slatopolsky, E., Caglar, S., Giadowska, L., Canterbury, J., Reiss, E. and Bricker, N. S., On the prevention of secondary hyperparathyroidism in experimental chronic renal disease using proportional reduction of dietary phosphate intake. *Kidney Int.*, 1972, **2**: 147.

Index

Index